THE UTTERMOST PARTS

SHORT STORIES ABOUT A MISSION TRIP TO AFRICA FEBRUARY 2012

Pam - Thank you for taking time to read my "stuff" and your encouraging words.
Linda
Matt. 28:19-20

BY

LINDA DERBY

ISBN 978-0-9847974-5-5
Softcover

Bible Translation is from the King James Version.

This book was printed in the United States of America.

To order additional copies of this book, contact:
Linda Derby
7247 N. 201 E. Ave.
Owasso, Ok 74055
918-398-840 H
918-521-3973
lindaderby@me.com

Published by
FWB Publications

TABLE OF CONTENTS

A Special thanks to Tina

All proceeds from book sales go to charity

Disclaimer: All stories are from the personal experiences of the author. The subject content is factual and in accordance to the writer's perception and understanding. Interpreters were used to translate the languages and every effort was made to keep the meaning of the language accurate and in agreement with those interviewed. The interpreters provided the spelling of the villages and individual names. Pictures are from personal collections and members of the team. Complete names of the team members and the name of the non-profit organization were not given in order to protect their privacy. No story or portion of a story may be used or copied without the permission of the author.

Biography

Linda Derby is an author, R.N., and a Healthcare Consultant. She is married and has three children and seven grandchildren. She is the author of the inspirational book, *Life's Sticky Wick* and the author of the biography, *His Story,* the true story about a POW from WWII.

She has co-authored the book, *Bismarck—Hometown U.S.A.*—a historical account of the town in Missouri where she grew up. She has numerous published articles in denominational magazines and has written numerous Christian plays and skits for performance. She has served as the Director of the Financial Aid Department at the California Christian College, Fresno, California; Founder and President of Bridge the Barriers Foundation, a nonprofit organization of the Harmony Church, Fresno, California; Co-founder and Director of the Hmong Bus Ministry, Harmony Church, Fresno, California, and has served as an educator of Hmong women and teenage girls.

Linda has served 25 years in church bus ministries in Missouri and California. She also has a lengthy career as an administrative nurse. Linda and her husband, Dr. Dale Derby, reside in Owasso, Oklahoma with two of their children and their families. She is an active member of the Rejoice Church where she is involved in the drama and music ministries.

**DEDICATED
TO
THE LADY IN PINK**

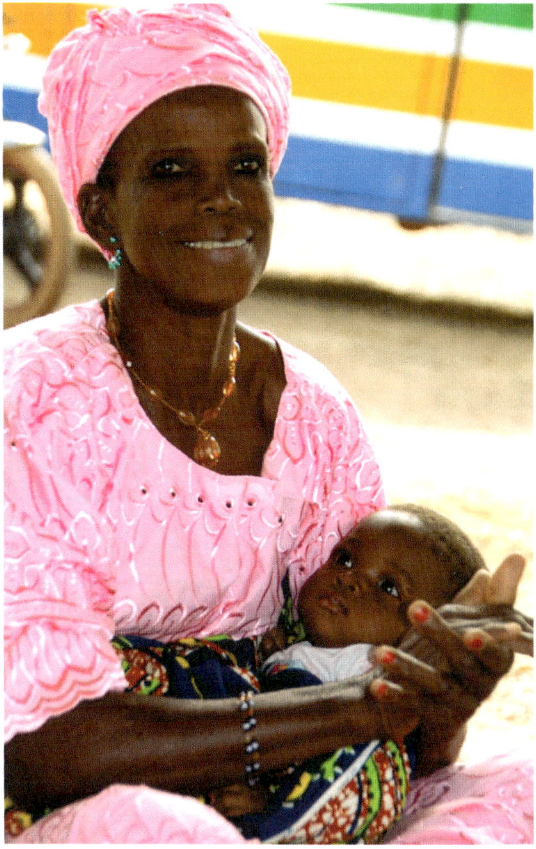

In God is my salvation and my glory: the rock of my strength, and my refuge is in God. (Psalm 62:7)

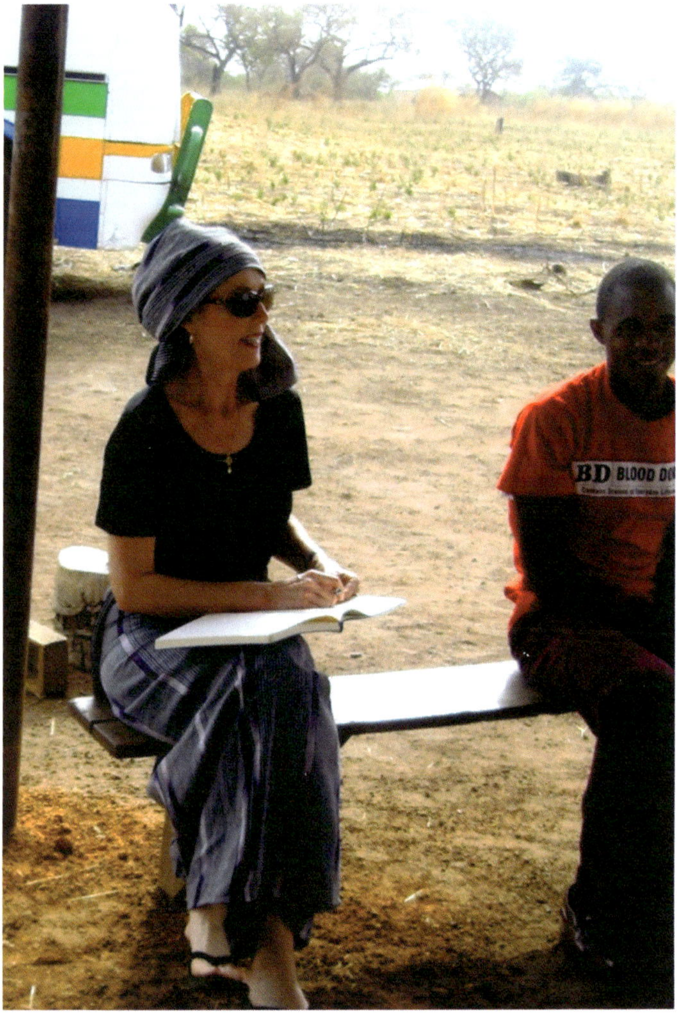

Linda Derby And Friend

INTRODUCTION

January 1, 2012

Time is fast approaching for our trip to Africa. I am excited on many levels and somewhat apprehensive. I have never been to Africa so I don't know what to expect. But I have been mentally and spiritually preparing for it ever since I realized I would definitely be going. I do not want to fill my head with expectations based on things I have already experienced from past reports of others. I want my head to be completely cleared—as a blank sheet of paper so that God can not only fill in the blanks, but also write the text. I want my senses filled with what God wants to teach and what God wants me to experience. I want my faith to come alive like never before. I want my heart feel what my eyes see. I want God to make it real all over again!

These are the words I journaled one evening as I was thinking about the soon approaching African trip my husband, son, and I would be making with a humanitarian organization that would construct or refurbish schools and churches for the community and deliver medical care to the people on the Ivory Coast. In some ways the words sound desperate and perhaps they were but I longed to "feel" my faith. I needed a refreshing—a spiritual awakening to burn bright once again. I wanted to witness the freshness of salvation as experienced by others. I wanted to see God work in a country that had been darkened by centuries of idolatry. I wanted to see God tear down the stronghold of Satan that had kept the people captive since the beginning of time. I needed a jolt and happily, God shook me and filled my senses as I asked with sights and sounds I knew were especially for me. He touched my heart in ways that were reminiscent to the joy I experienced the day of my salvation so many years ago.

I was touched by the determination of the African believers—their peace and contentment in spite of their surroundings and conditions. I was in awe with how they praised God and danced to please Him. They were happy and so excited about their faith and what God had done for them. My spirit was refreshed with what I saw and heard and I left with a great sense of gratitude that God is God over all and can be found even in the darkest places in Africa. My heart truly felt what my eyes saw and as many have said, "the trip was a life-changing experience."

I wrote about some of the people and places I visited during the trip. It was my intention to share with others the workings of God and perhaps they too would be blessed by the faithfulness of a loving Father to His children.

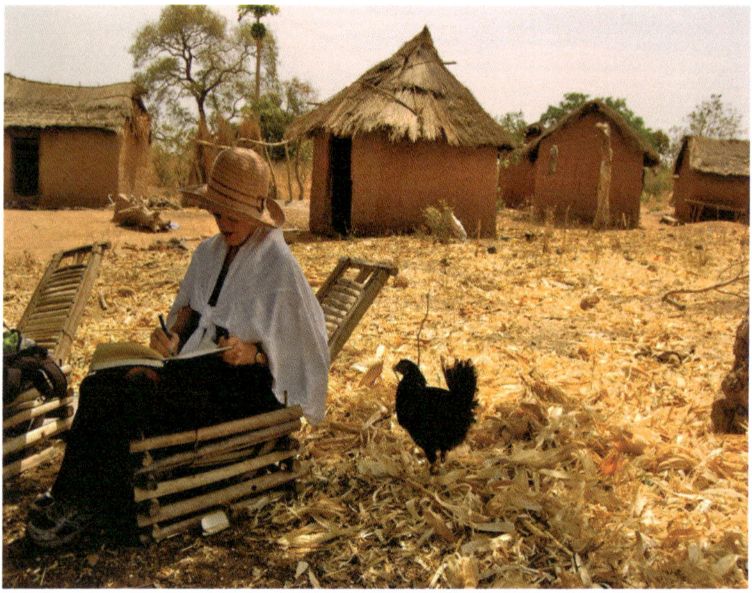

GOD WILL MAKE A WAY WHEN THERE SEEMS TO BE NO WAY

The title of this story is also the name of a popular praise and worship song by Don Moen. Our group's song leader, Bruce, would sing this song quite often before our morning devotions while visiting "Camp" Doropo. It had a catchy little tune that you might find yourself humming over and over during the wee hours of night. The title also served as the question I asked God as our wound team ventured into the African villages. My heart was broken by what I saw—the poverty, oppression, hopelessness. I asked myself, how will God, how could God possibly make a way for them?

It was a hot Monday morning. Bob was our team leader and would be driving the van into the villages for the wound care team to treat those in need. Making the trip that day were Blaine, Allen, Christina, Sara, myself, an Ivorian Pastor we called Pastor Abel, an interpreter, and a guide by the name of Eli. We left camp around 9:00 a.m. and drove approximately 35 minutes on the roughest road I had ever been on! Thirty-five minutes actually seemed like an eternity. Travel was slow because of the potholes in the road. The potholes were the size of houses. With my bad back, I quickly learned how to brace myself so as not to be injured by the sudden disappearance of the vehicle into the mouth of the deep pit. When I felt the bottom drop out of the road, I would brace myself using both hands and suspend myself in midair until the vehicle resurfaced and the seat bounced up to meet my bottom. It worked well.

The village was difficult to locate. Bob stopped the van at some unknown destination and told everyone that we needed to get out and walk to the village. Our guide could not tell us how far we would need to walk but indicated the village was down the road (path) a ways. I am told that most Africans have no concept of time or distance. Down the road could mean 100 yards or ten miles.

The guide (Eli) started walking on the narrow dusty path. The younger members of our group followed while the older members brought up the rear. I followed Pastor Abel toward the end and Bob followed me as we ventured into unknown territory in search of the village.

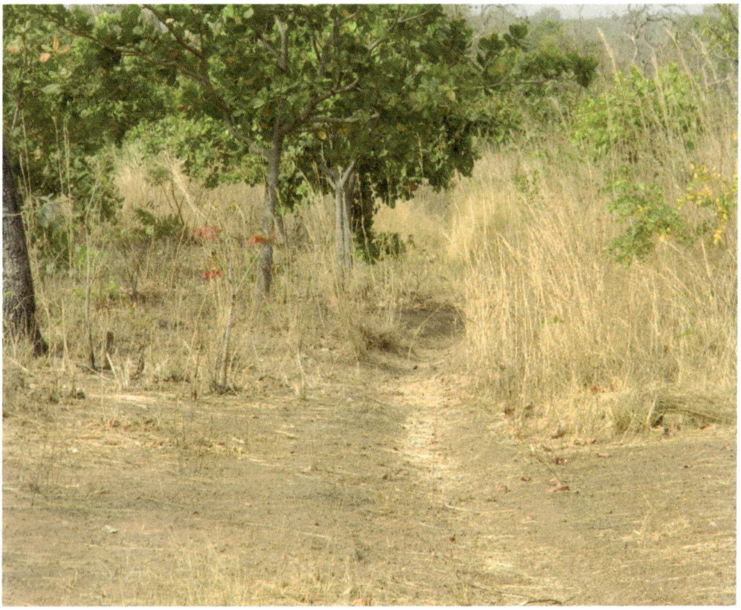

The Path Leading To The Lost Village.

The heat from the African sun was intense. It was at least 90 degrees and there was no breeze to cool things down. We hiked about 25 minutes or around two miles. I became extremely hot during this time and kept thinking when would we get to the village. I started humming the tune of "God will make a way" while asking God to please show us the way off the path to the village! God must have been talking to Bob because suddenly Bob made a decision to turn around. He told the guide he did not want to lead the team on a journey without some knowledge of where the village was located. The guide insisted it was still just down the road. Bob insisted we turn around and we did.

I made the comment to Bob that at least the journey back to the van would be downhill. He laughed and said, "We have been walking downhill since we left the van!" I thought he was kidding but he wasn't. I followed Pastor Abel as we began the trek back. I took more time to look at the surroundings as I walked. The path was wide enough for one person and the path was well worn. In some places, the path was flanked on both sides by grass taller than myself. An occasional baobab tree could be seen. These trees were quite unique looking without their leaves. They appeared to be growing upside down. From a distance, the tree looked as if it had it's "head" stuck in the ground with a complex root system sticking out from the top reaching to the sky. The tree was really different.

Children would suddenly appear along the path. They must have been playing in the weeds and grasses and saw us as we walked back toward the van. They seemed to be happy with smiling faces. Several of us stopped to say hello and shook their hands. They wanted to touch us. I suppose they don't see many light skinned people and we probably were a curiosity.

Some of the children were sick with parasites. Their bloated bellies attested to that. Other children had coughs and runny noses. All were dirty as would be expected. There were no paved roads or sidewalks to walk or play on. None wore shoes. They were scantily dressed and the younger ones were naked. They had no choice but to be dirty.

As I followed Pastor Abel I observed several things: He was very familiar with walking dusty, dirt paths. His sandaled feet bore evidence to this. His heels were thick and calloused and his dark skin was very dry. Evidence of many years of wear and tear doing what he was called to do—telling others about the Good News of Jesus Christ. He also did not complain about the heat or the fact we could not initially find the village. He was on a mission. He just kept walking while taking long strides to get to his destination. He reminded me of the disciples who Christ commissioned and gave power to go preach the Kingdom of

God to the villages and cities, while healing diseases, and having all authority over the devils. Pastor Abel was one of them—a true disciple.

The four-mile round trip "stress test" was finally over. We all passed and made it back to the van. We boarded and turned our vehicle around and headed back into the direction we came. We stopped the van just a short distance from the original stop. There was a village that sat back from the road just a bit. Someone made the decision that this was the village we were to visit!

Many young children greeted us as we got off the van. They were excited to see us and we were excited to see them. Children are children everywhere. They made me smile by their enthusiasm. I fell in love with all of them and that was when God started speaking to my heart.

My husband and I spent over 25 years in bus ministry working with children so much like these—innocent, sweet, precious children in the sight of God who would one day know right from wrong and would need a Savior. I immediately connected with them and wanted to teach them some vital English words like—"Jesus loves me this I know; for the Bible tells me so." But I couldn't stay there playing with the children because the team had to first meet the chief of the village to get permission to do wound care and preach the Good News. This was a function we were obligated to do at every village in order to carry out what God called us to do.

We walked a short distance to a large tree located in the center of the village. Pastor Abel and the interpreter went to work asking to speak with the chief of the village. Before the chief arrived, several men brought chairs for us to sit on. They also shook our hands but would not make eye contact with us while shaking our hands. They also shook our hand in an unusual way by placing their left hand on their right forearm as they shook our hand. This was their way to express a very special welcome to the village.

The chief emerged from his hut carrying a stick to aid his walking. He was wearing a pair of pink-laced women's Capri pants! He also wore a Red Cross cap and a long sleeved brown and gray shirt. He shook hands with each of the team members and then sat down with us under the tree. His eyes captivated me. They were dark, dark, brown but very warm and kind. I could tell that behind those eyes were many stories of what he had seen and experienced in the many years on this earth.

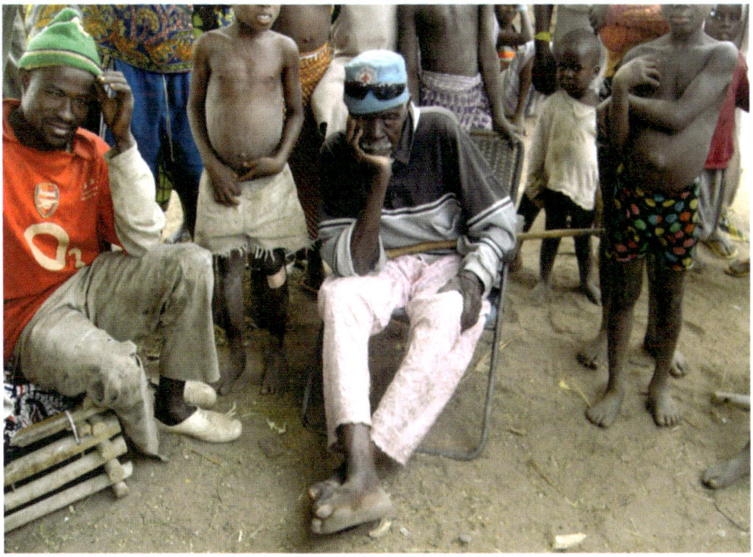

The Village Chief

Pastor Abel and the interpreter began speaking to the chief in Lobi about why we were there. The pastor told the chief we would offer them the Good News of Jesus Christ and then help heal their wounds. The chief was agreeable to that. Then the interpreter took a megaphone and called the villagers to come meet under the tree. With this announcement, a breeze blew through the village as a welcome relief for the hot and the weary.

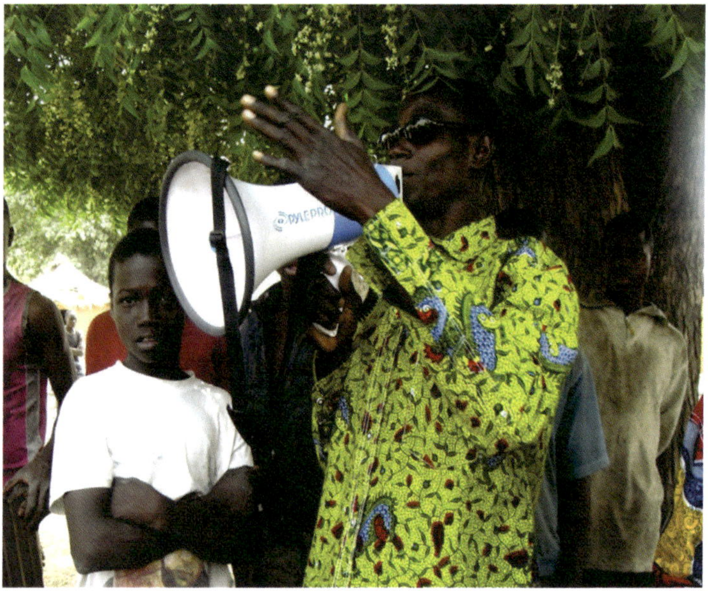

The Call To Worship

While waiting for the villagers to assemble under the tree, I took advantage of the few minutes to just observe. There were mothers nursing babies, children playing everywhere, crippled people with sad faces, older adults sitting in chairs or on the dirt, and women carrying large objects and baskets on their heads. There were also large metal pots sitting on the dirt outside their huts. Pots are a sign of wealth. The more pots you own, the wealthier the family.

Reality soon made its presence known. This was not a Christian village. There were signs of fetish gods they worshiped. Sticks placed in the ground holding dried out gourds stood in the center of the village and in the fields. Some huts had these sticks placed by the door. Children wore beads around their waists with colorful string for protection. These amulets were to ward-off bad luck or evil.

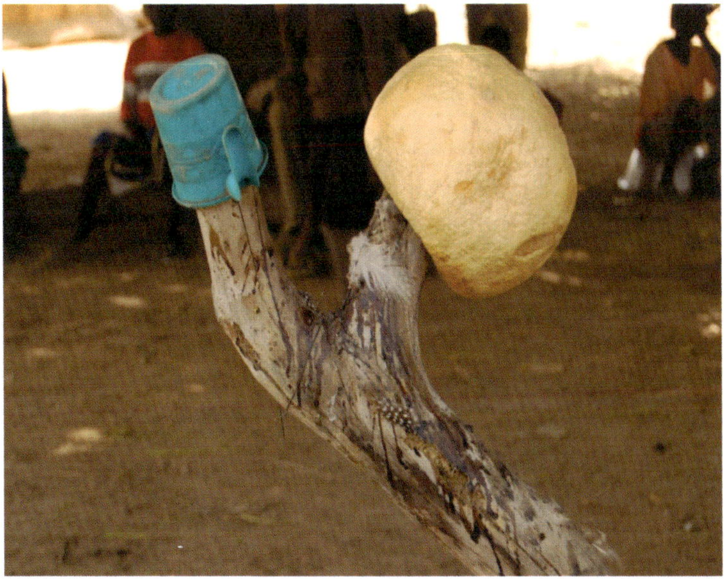

(Notice the dried blood of the sacrifice on the limb.)
Signs Of Fetish Worship

I was reminded of the Hmong ministry my husband and I were involved with while living in California. Their cultural religion/fetishes are very similar. They are primarily animists. They believe anything can be a god. They also "worship" the devil or DA but not out of respect but out of fear of being punished by the devil. They used all kinds of amulets as protection against evil including feathers or dried bones attached over the doorpost of their houses, sticks standing in the yard, and colorful string tied around the wrists. Some parents even disguised their young children as flowers in order to keep evil out of their homes. Considering all that must be believed or practiced in these fetish religions, it would appear that Christianity would be so much easier to accept—but I know this was not the case.

The villagers began to appear under the tree. There were approximately 30 adults present with more men than women. Of course, children were ever present. Pastor Abel asked our team to pray that it would not be difficult for the people to believe. Blaine led in prayer followed by Allen. These people have so much to overcome just to believe. Their cultural fetishes and the hardships they endure just staying alive. I once read a book by a Christian pastor who believed that the lower levels of human needs (food, shelter, clothing, security, etc.) must first be met before a person becomes a ready candidate to accept Christ. I can see his point. How many of these villagers have enough food to eat, or proper shelter, clothing, or security of any kind not to mention overcoming fetish beliefs and fears of the devil? Missionaries certainly have a hard row to hoe but this is not to discount the power of God and His ability to change the hardest heart and do the impossible. I am reminded that God's ways are not my ways and His thinking is certainly not my thinking. God is so awesome!

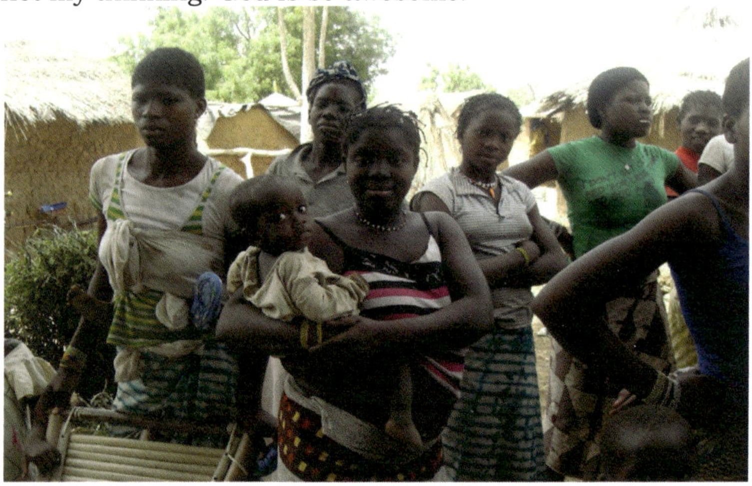

The Villagers Assembling To Hear The Good News

Pastor Abel began preaching. The chief listened intently as did others sitting close by. I soon realized I was witnessing the Good News being shared for the very first time to people living in the 21st century. This was a hard concept to embrace. Then the pastor moved closely to the chief. His message was being directed to him. I suppose that if a chief accepts Christ, so goes the village. The pastor ended his message and the people applauded.

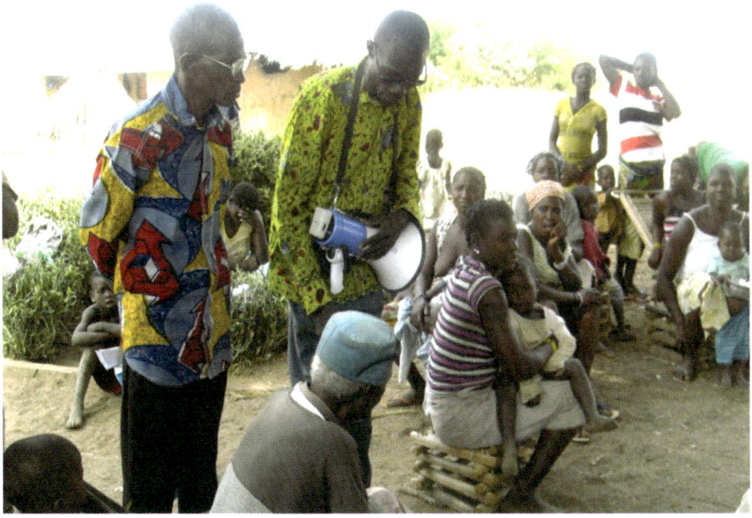

Pastor Abel, The Interpreter, And The Village Chief Discussing The Good News.

Pastor Abel continued to speak to the adults while the team started wound care. I hung around the team for a while just to see what injuries were being treated. I am an R.N. but I did not want to work in that capacity on the trip. I wanted my heart to be ready to receive what God was telling me. My goal was to write and only interject my medical opinion if needed or asked.

The little ones had scrapes and cuts that could easily turn into life-threatening infections and sepsis. They could lose a limb or their life by a "simple" infection. We take so much for granted living in the United States that allows us to have appropriate antibiotics on hand, clean bandages, and access to doctors to keep us healthy. We hardly think twice about a cut or an abrasion. We know we will heal and suffer no consequences.

Some villagers had fungal infections and some had embedded objects under the skin that had been there for quite some time. We were unable to lance and remove foreign objects in the field. One man had pain in his palm when he moved his thumb. It looked like something was rolling under his skin as he moved his thumb. This most likely was a ruptured tendon that needed surgery to repair. Obviously, we were unable to do anything for him while on the field. He would need to go to the hospital for treatment.

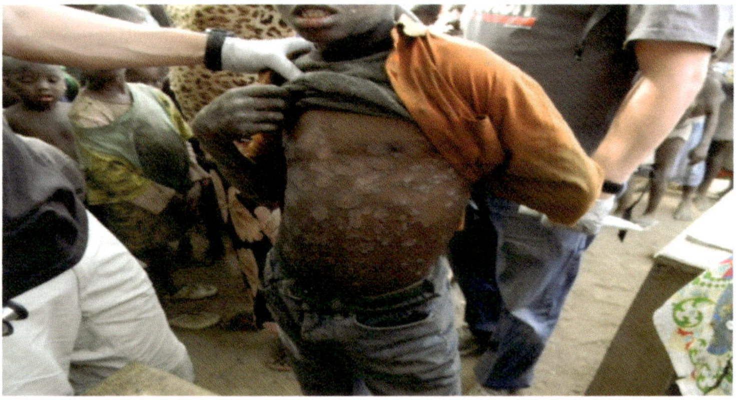

Child With Fungal Infection Of The Skin

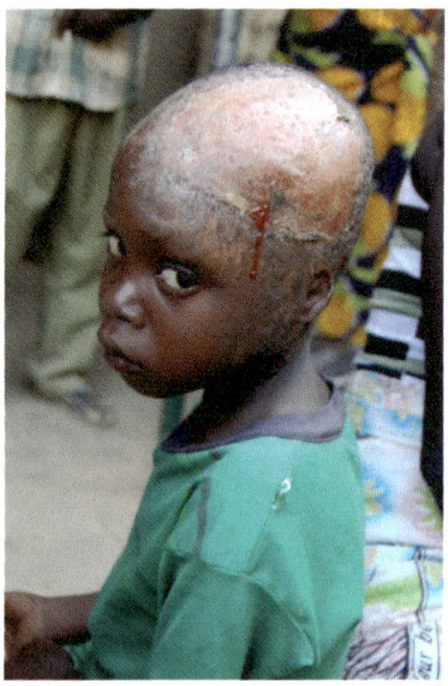

Child With Infection From Burned Scalp

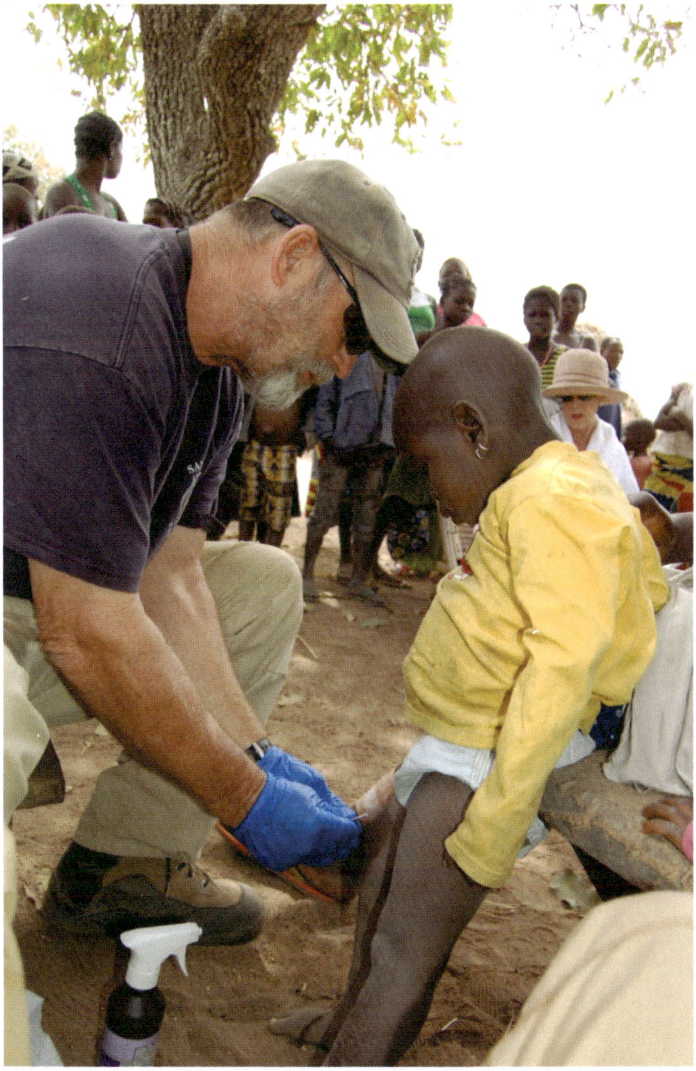

**Bob, Our Team Leader,
Giving Wound Care To A Young Villager.**

One young lady sat on the stool to be treated by the team. She had a deep gash on her left leg. Blaine said these are the wounds "we like to see." He gently cleaned the wound and then prayed over it asking God to heal the wound completely. The woman calmly sat on the stool nursing her baby as he dressed her leg.

Wound care continued for approximately one hour. Pastor Abel was still talking with the adult villagers. Blaine began to play with the children, as did Christina and Sara. Blaine made a noise with his lips to the tune of "Jesus Loves Me." The kids loved it and started clapping their hands. Then Blaine started dancing with the children. A couple of the girls did the Lobi dance. This dance looked like a physical impossibility. It looked as if every vertebra moved in opposite directions at the same time. It also looked painful but everyone liked the entertainment.

I needed a few moments by myself to reflect on our visit. I walked toward the other side of the "town square" to be alone but I was soon followed by about 30 children. I decided to take advantage of the time and continue to teach them the words of "Jesus Loves Me" and then sing the song to them. I knew they would try to sing the song back to me because they mimicked everything. I gathered them around to face me and I slowly recited the words to the song. They repeated the words not knowing what they were saying let alone knowing anything about Jesus. Then I began to sing the song to them one line at a time. The children began to sing after me. When I heard their voices, I thought the angels had descended from heaven. Their beautiful little voices were pitch perfect and they were singing about Jesus they knew not. I could only sing through the song one time as I was overcome with emotion. I started to pray. I closed my eyes and extended my hands over the children and I tearfully asked God, how would these children find the way to Him when things are so stacked against them. How could they know the Jesus they had sung about?

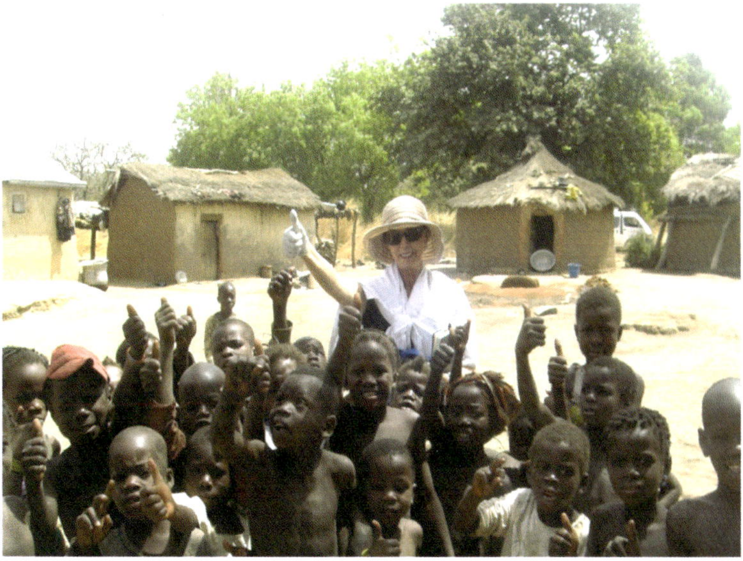

Village Children With Linda

My heart was broken. The only hope for these villagers was Jesus and the spiritual warfare between good and evil within their community was great. Who would win?

The team was walking towards me and I realized it was time to get back on the van and go to the next village. I said good-bye to the children and told them not to forget that Jesus loved them. God would have to do the interpretation in their hearts for them to understand what I had said. As I boarded the van, I asked Eli if any of the villagers accepted Christ. He said four adult men accepted Christ but not the chief. I asked if any pastor made follow-up visits to these new converts. Eli said that Pastor Abel wrote down the names of the new believers so he could revisit them in the future. My heart jumped for joy.

God spoke to my heart as we were traveling to the next village. He reminded me of my earlier question I had asked while walking on the dusty path—I wanted Him to show us the way to the village and He did. He reminded me of my questions in the village regarding the children and how would He make a way for them to know Jesus. Then it hit me. The new converts in the village would be the catalyst. From the dusty path into the village, into the hearts of the new believers—God had made a way for those children and other villagers to know Jesus by the testimonies and witness of the new believers! God had made a way for those precious, innocent children. They now had hope and one day, I am convinced they will know the Jesus they had sung about. Praise God!

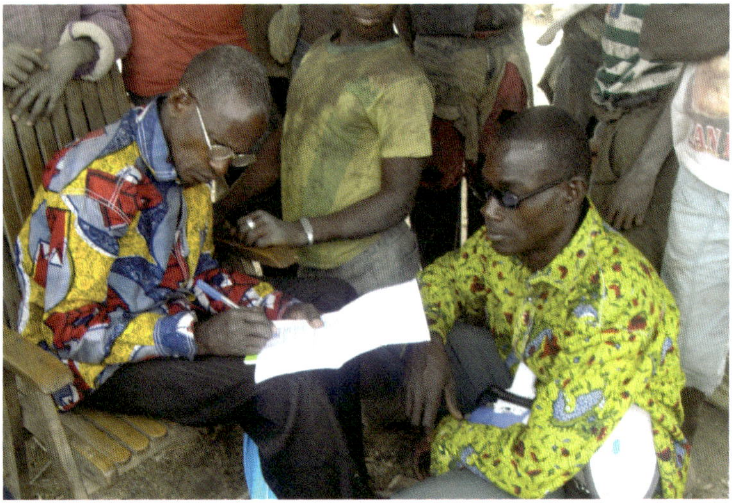

Pastor Abel Recording The Names Of New Believers.

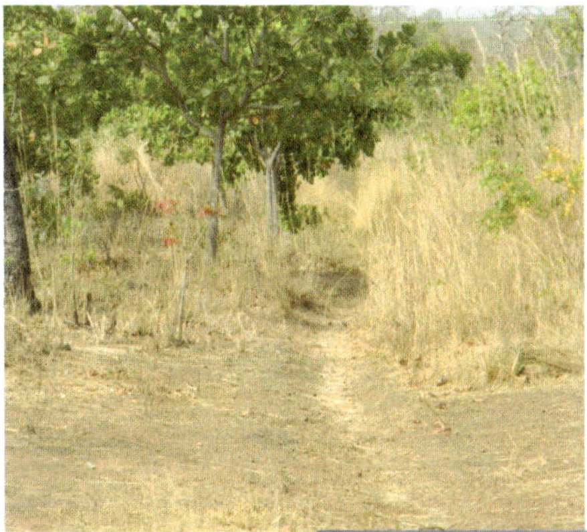

From the path . . .

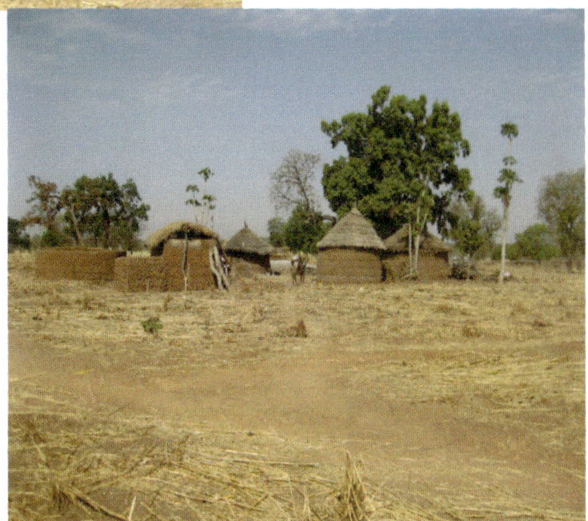

To the village . . .

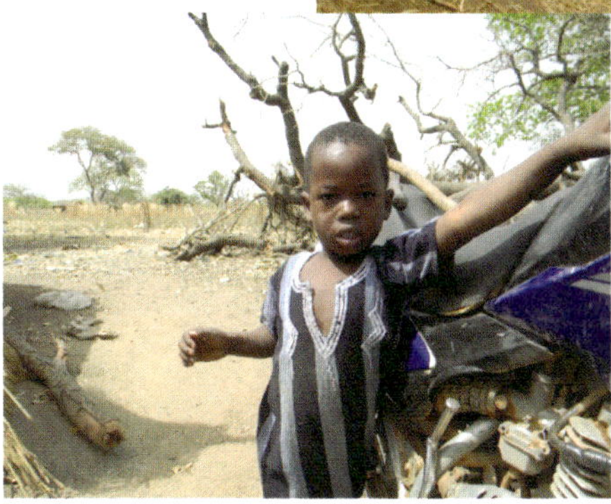

To the hearts of the people, God will make a way . . .

Our visit to this village can best be summed-up from the words of the song by Don Moen:

God will make a way when there seems to be no way.
He works in ways we cannot see
He will make a way for me
He has been my guide
Holds me closely to His side
With love and strength for each new day
He will make a way
He will make a way

A WOMAN NAMED ADELAIDE

I spent the first three days of our stay at Camp Doropo working 15-hour shifts in Post-op care. This was quite the experience. We were giving patient care in a very primitive setting without the conveniences of modern hospitals. Post-op was located in a large rectangular tent with an open-flapped door at each end and similar windows on the sides of the tent. This was our ventilation and air conditioning system assisted by a box fan sitting on the Post-op floor. The open doors also served as our only light source for a day or so. Flashlights were used at night until our construction crew rigged-up some lighting. As appreciative as we were for the fan and the bright light of the sun, the tent was extremely hot!

Chaise lounge chairs served as cots. Fourteen of these cots lined the inner walls with an occasional curtain to separate the men from women. The facility required frequent sweeping of the dirt that blew in from the wind or tracked in by the many family members of the patients. Many of the patients we received from the OR should have been in an ICU with proper monitoring and appropriate equipment. Overall, things went well because God was in it!

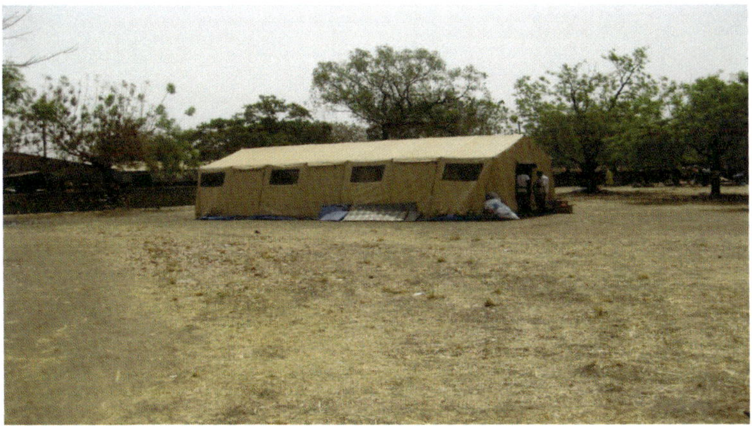

Post-Op Tent

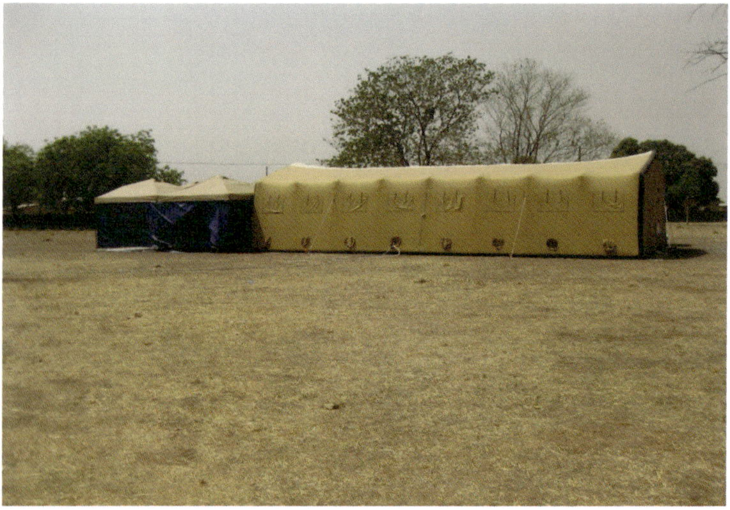

Mobile Surgical Unit

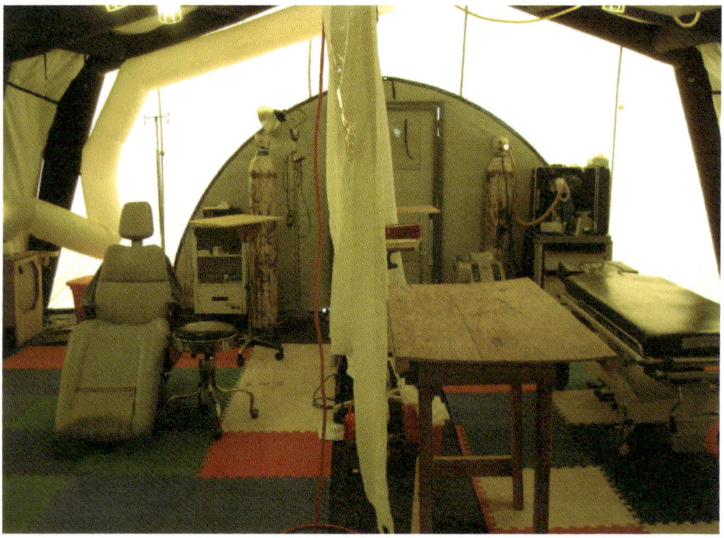

Interior Of Mobile Surgical Unit
The Area Where Oral/Maxillary Surgery And General Surgery Was Performed

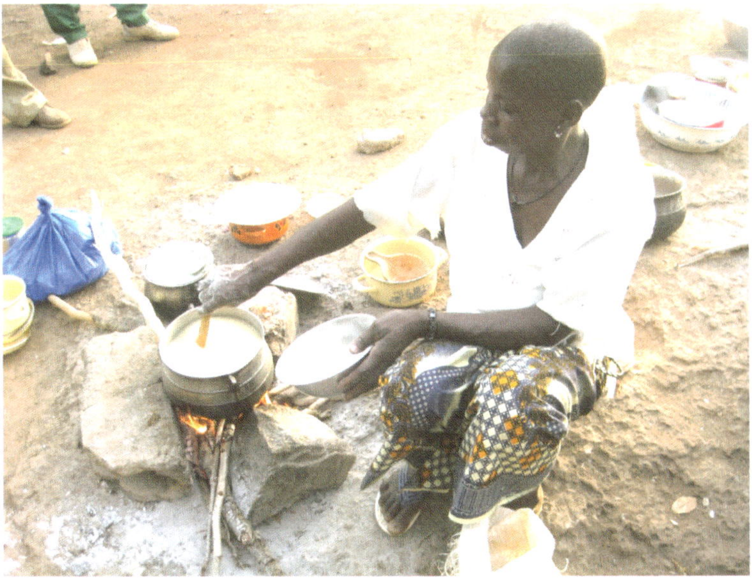

Cooking For A Hospitalized Family Member

Another nurse, Jamie, and I took care of the patients that were admitted to Post-op. We established some routine about the activity inside the tent. There was also an interpreter by the name of Binni who stayed in the tent most of the time. He is actually the young man in charge of the school in Doropo. He was a very nice young man and extremely helpful as an interpreter.

We saw many serious Post-op cases. One young boy in particular received major maxillary-facial surgery and had some bones removed from his jaw and mouth. He came back to Post-op with a huge dressing on the side of his face. The entire left side of his face was extremely swollen to the size of a soft ball. He looked absolutely miserable but did not complain of pain until six hours after surgery. The African people have a high tolerance to pain.

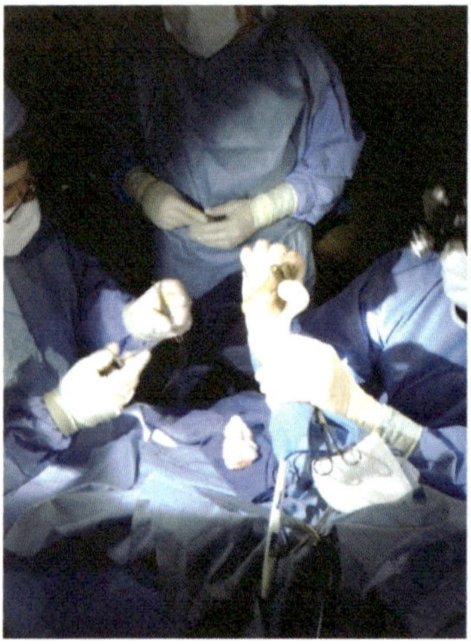

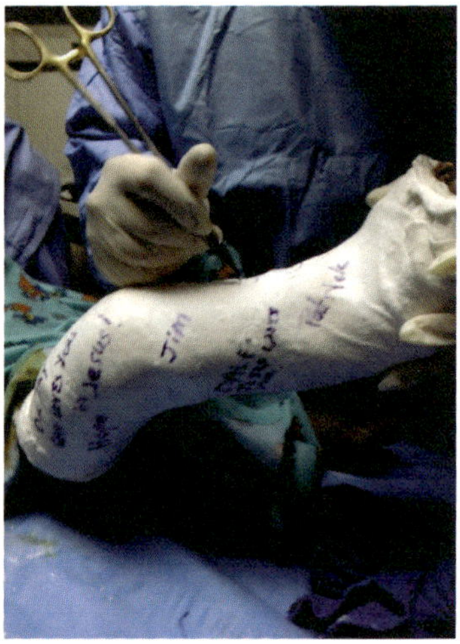

Scenes From The Operating Room

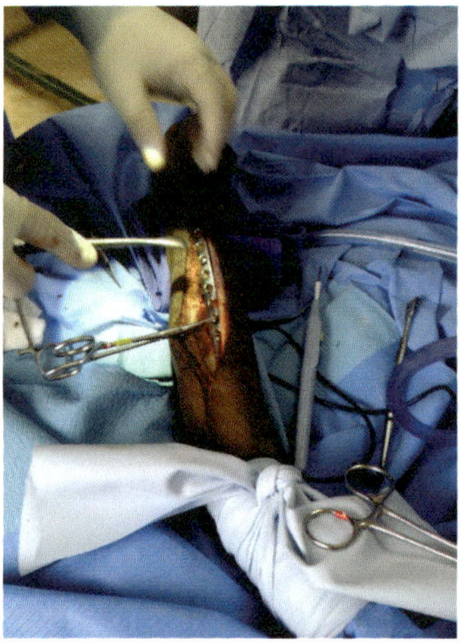

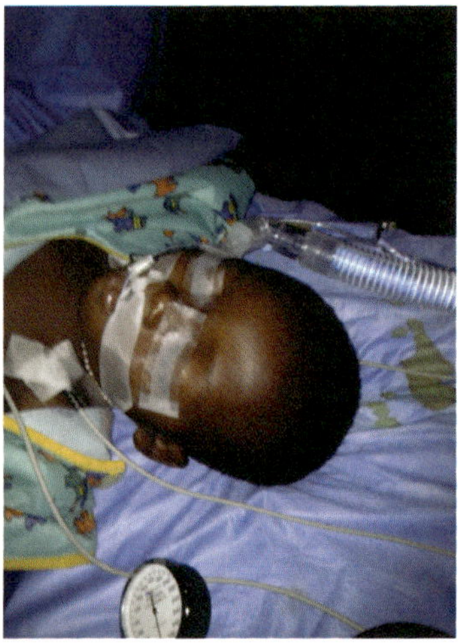

There was an OB/GYN doctor that joined the medical team this year. He was an excellent doctor who performed many surgeries on women who were very ill with multiple diseases. The patients would come back to Post-op after having major surgery with the only pain medicine ordered—plain Tylenol or Ibuprofen! I thought to myself—why even bother? Most people require an extra strength Tylenol or Ibuprofen for a slight headache but not abdominal surgery. We needed Demerol or Morphine. Occasionally we could give the patient IV or IM Nubain for pain but this was given sparingly. This is not to degrade the excellence of the physician. I am sure he would have given stronger pain medication if the medication were available. We gave what medications we had and did the best we could while performing under conditions that would have closed down any hospital in America. The Africans were greatly appreciative of our efforts.

We did lose one patient. She was very sick with cervical cancer, endometriosis, and other associated female problems. She was my patient initially but she crashed about an hour after receiving her in Post-op. She was taken back to the OR and the doctor reopened her surgical incision. She had bled internally and her abdomen was full of blood. After many hours trying to save the woman, she died. The doctor later told me that once he reopened the patient he discovered additional life threatening problems. He said the woman would have most likely died even in the ideal setting of an American hospital. Her death left a dark cloud over the camp but there was some good news that chased the cloud away. Mike, our camp leader, told us she was a believer! He said something to the effect that considering all that was wrong with her—how much better off she was in the presence of God and would not have to go back to all of this. (Indicating the palatial life of an African woman.)

Jamie left the Post-op area to assist the doctors in the OR when our patient crashed. I remained in the Post-op to care for the other patients. Things were quiet and the patients were comfortable. It was then I noticed a young woman sitting on her bedside who had abdominal surgery the previous day. She was reading her Bible. I asked Binni to go with me so I might talk with her.

I sat on the cot next to her. I told her my name and asked what name she was called. There were two first names given on her medical record. She said it was Adelaide even though she did not pronounce it like it was spelled. I asked what she was reading. She told Binni she was reading the 26th Psalm and then pointed to it. I asked if she minded me sharing with her the 23rd Psalm. She smiled and said she would like that. I asked Binni to begin reading the 23rd Psalm. When he finished, I told her that with Jesus we have no wants. He supplies all our needs if we follow Him. He brings comfort and rest when we are weak and weary. He restores our soul with healing and encouragement and will guide our path as we walk through life. One day when we pass through the valley of the shadow of death, He will be there right beside us. We do not have to fear anything even the attacks of Satan. He fights for us constantly. He gives us mercy when we do wrong and brings joy and peace to our lives. And one day when this life is over here on earth, are spirit will join Him in heaven and live with Him forever.

I prayed for her then that God would meet her needs and heal her body and restore her health. I prayed that she might stay strong in faith and determined to live her life that would draw others to Him.

After the prayer, Adelaide smiled really big and thanked me. The woman on the cot next to her smiled and thanked me for the sharing of God's Word. She too was a believer. Adelaide then asked how I spelled my name because she wanted to name her baby after me. I was honored.

It started out as a bad day in Post-op but was made brighter with the sharing of God's Word with another believer—a believer so different from me yet so similar because we shared the common thread of salvation through Jesus Christ.

SUNDAY—A DAY OF REST

After three long, hot, work intensive days in the Post-op, I was grateful that Sunday had arrived. We campers were given a choice where we could attend church—the church in town or board the bus and go into the village. I chose the village.

Approximately 50 people boarded the bus to go to the village. It was the village where our group had built a church last year. (I regret I did not get the name of the village.) We American women dressed-up in Lobi garb and wore long wrap-around skirts and headpieces. We left camp around 8:00 a.m. and drove through Doropo. All eyes were on the sights of the city.

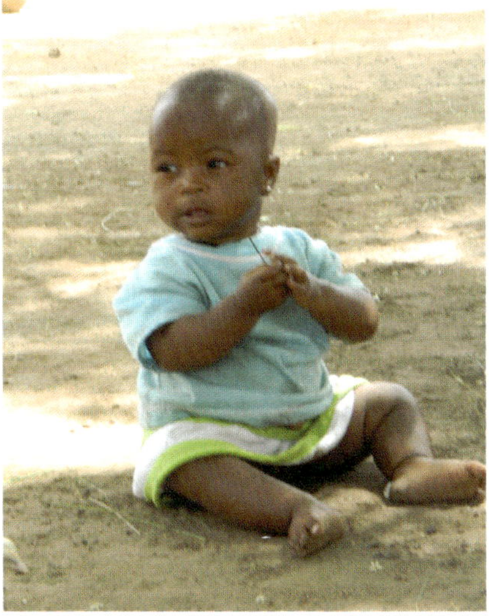

Is There Hope For This Child?

Unbelievable poverty! Filth wouldn't quite describe the situation. There were barefoot children playing on trash heaps that dotted the landscape everywhere. Men were lounging around at storefronts and other social places. There were many stores opened for business but I was not sure what they were selling. I did notice some type of food stand that had raw meat laid out on a rack in the open air, exposed to the sun and flying varmints. I could not imagine anyone actually buying and eating that stuff! I saw nothing modern or new throughout the town. There were some discards of modernization left by possibly visitors from other countries but nothing new.

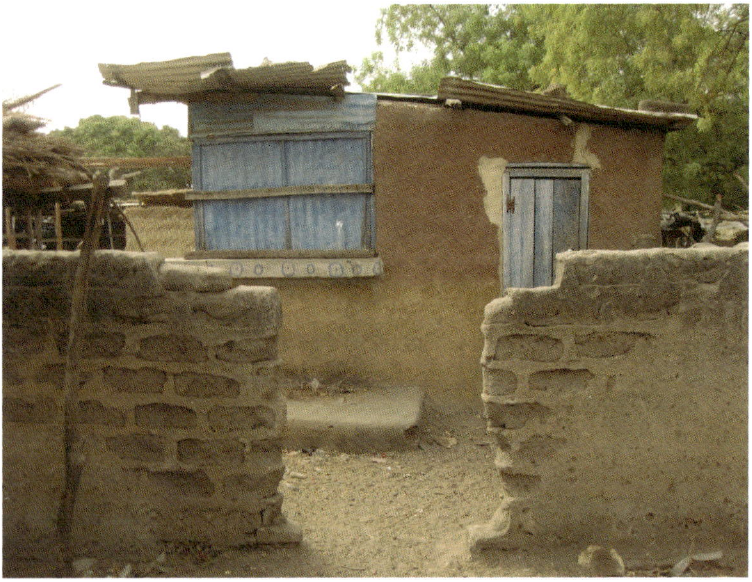

A Family Dwelling In Doropo

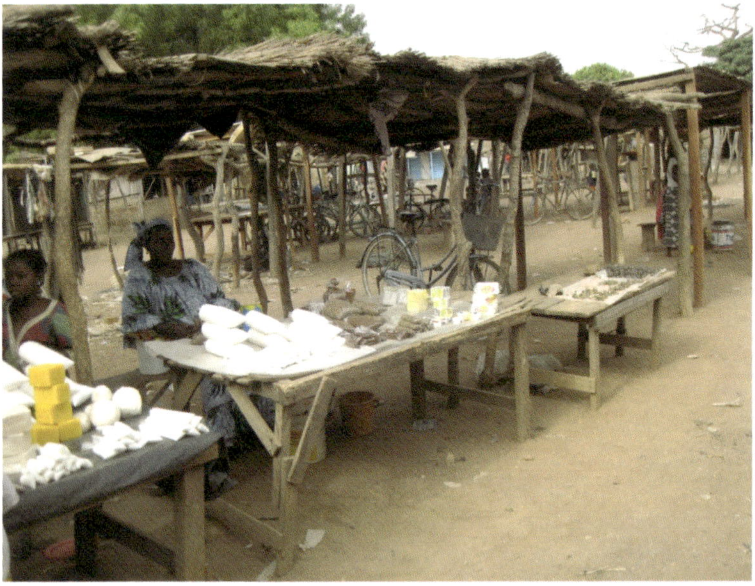

The Market

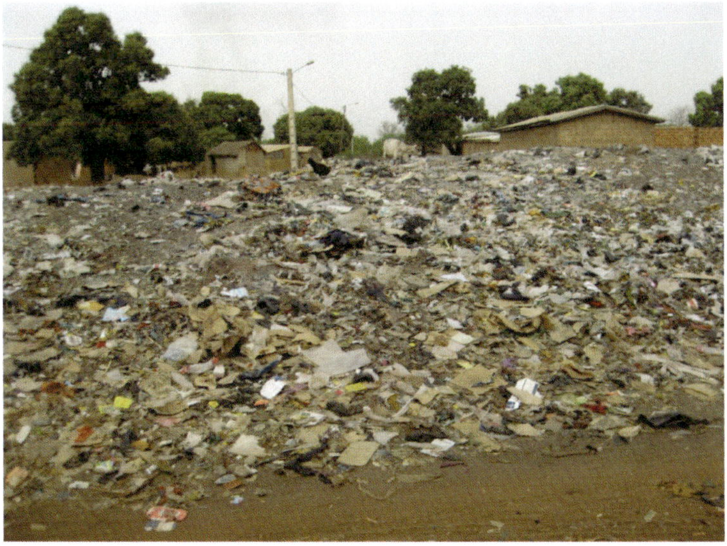

One Of Many Trash Heaps Inside Of Town.

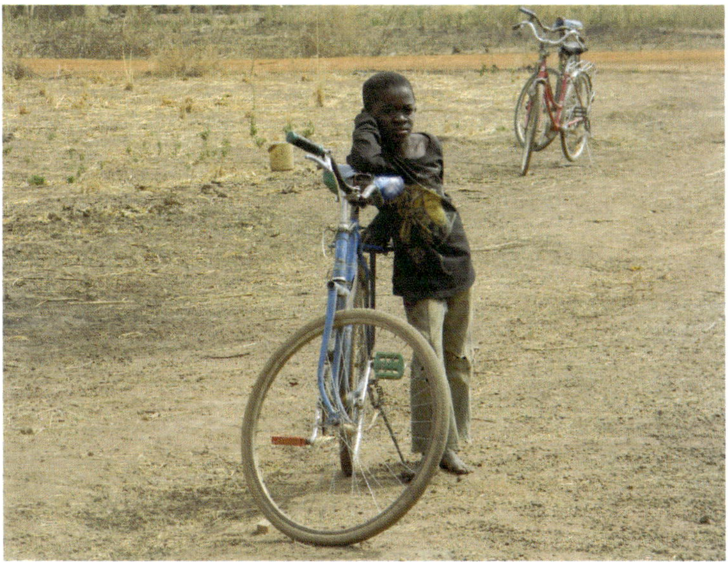

Young Resident Of Doropo

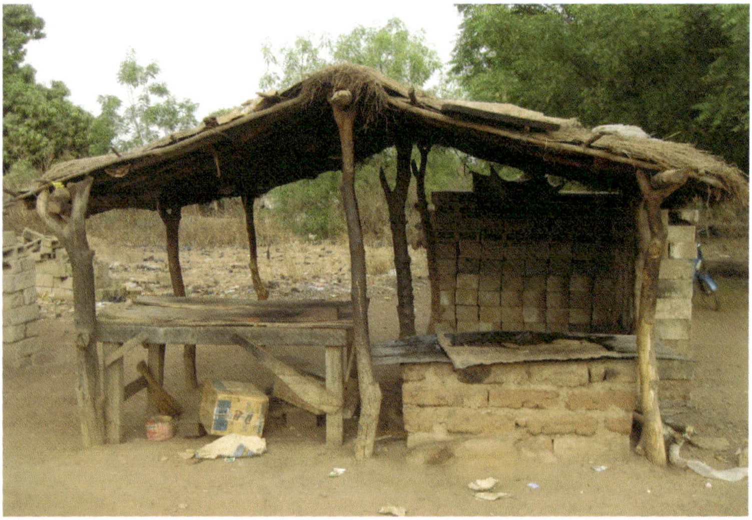

A Business Dwelling

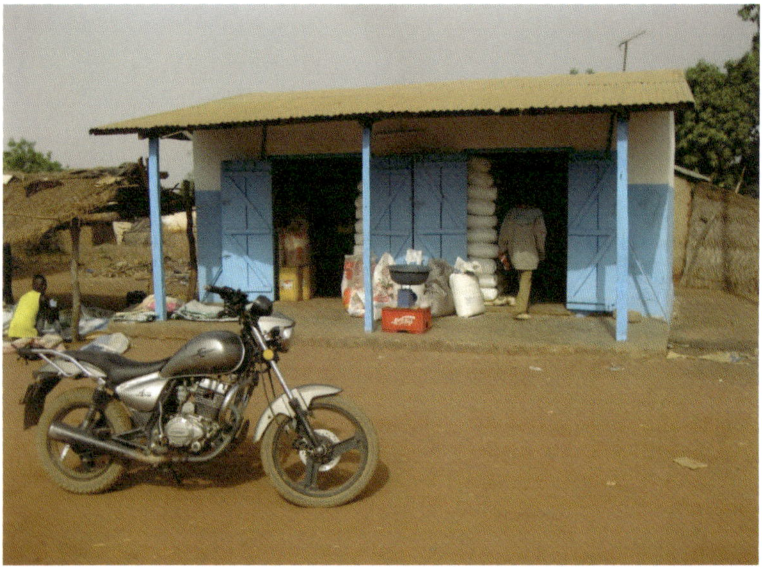

The General Store

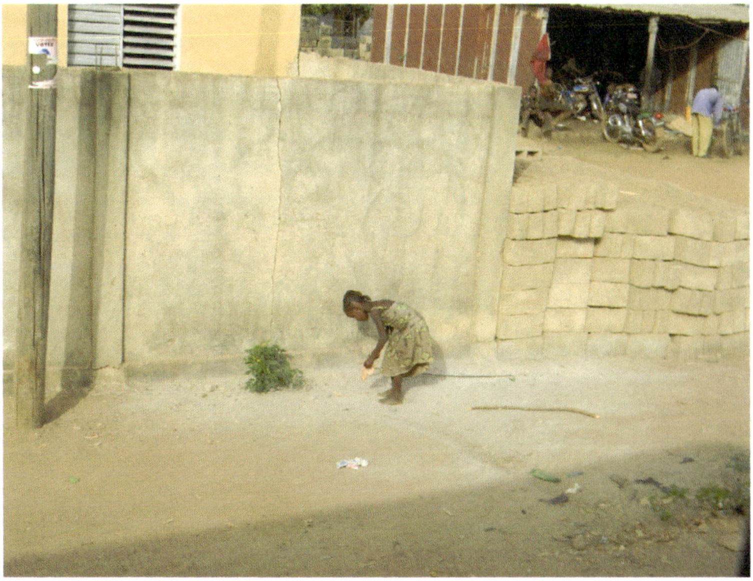

Children Of Doropo

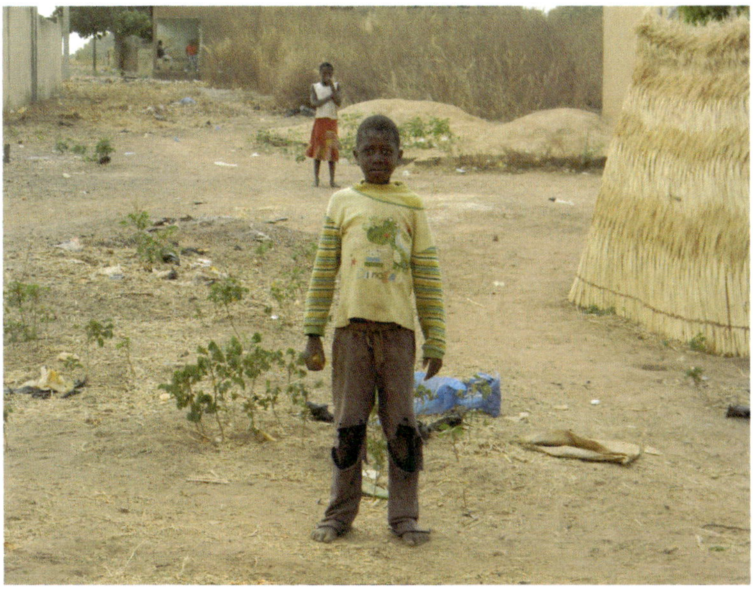

We were leaving town and on the right side of the road was a mansion. It was a huge home surrounded by a solid wall, with beautiful landscaping and I am told, a swimming pool on the grounds. This place belonged to some government official. The wealthy government official lived like a king with all the conveniences of modern technology while his subjects lived in abject poverty. Such a contrast! How could anyone with so much live with himself when he looked out his upstairs air-conditioned bedroom window and saw the inequality around him, most likely caused by his government.

As we left the town, I started to observe the nature in this part of Africa. The countryside was pretty but in a rugged way. There was an absence of mature trees that I did not expect. I later heard that most of the tall mature trees were harvested for wood several years ago. Only a few remained. The dirt was red-brown and it was obvious that volcanic activity once reigned supreme. Large lava rock could be seen above the earth's surface as well as granite rock. Everything was covered with red-brown dust and looked dirty. Cotton was grown and harvested in this part of Africa and some families had small, irrigated green gardens. If it was not irrigated, it was brown.

Yam mounds could often be seen growing in large clumps above the ground. Yams resembled the sweet potato but were much larger. Village farmers grow yams to provide starch or filler for their diets but they do not provide substantial nutrients for good health. Women will beat the yam into a starchy substance called futu and then will serve it to her family.

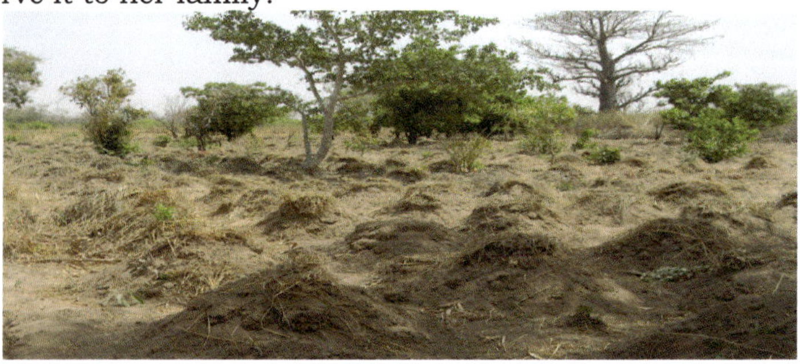

Yam Mounds

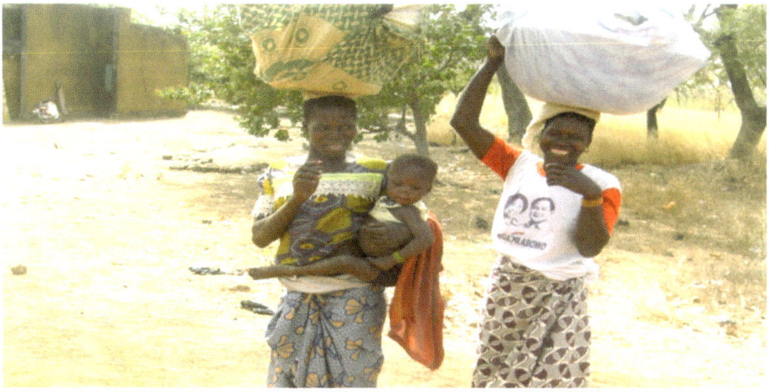

Ladies With Their Daily Chores

On our way to the next village for church, we passed several women carrying large pots and baskets on their heads while holding a baby in her arms or packing one on her back. What A Life!

There were large termite mounds scattered about the countryside. They resembled large sand castles children make at the beach. Someone said that if a woman gave birth to a baby and if something was wrong with the child, i.e. weakness, deformity, etc., the mother would put the baby in a termite mound and leave it. The mother would return the next day to the termite mound and if the baby was still alive, she took the baby home. I supposed if the baby lived the mother believed it was strong enough to survive. What a horrible practice!

We finally arrived at the church. It was an open structure that looked like an Oklahoma pole barn. Several villagers had already arrived along with the pastor, the village chief and his brother. Some´ (pronounced So May) was also present. Some´ was a Christian, a nurse, interpreter, and many other useful things. He had traveled to the United States and was a good friend to Mike our camp leader and the Free Will Baptist missionaries who once lived in the area. He was invaluable to us during our visit. God had used him mightily as a missionary to his people.

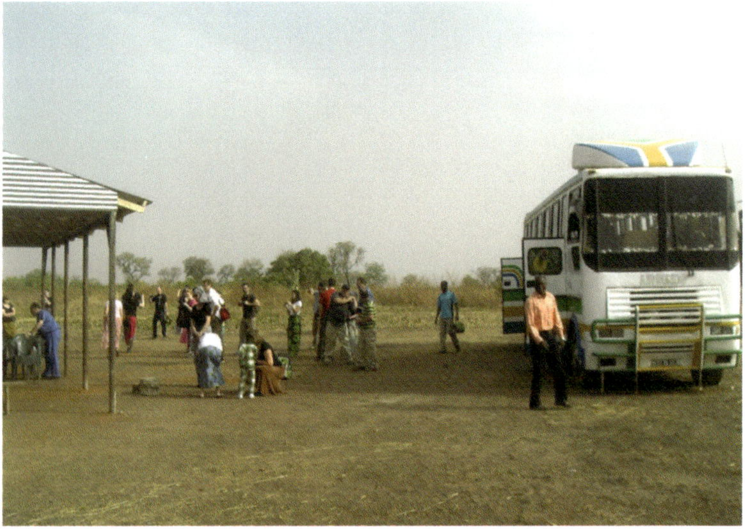

Arriving At Church

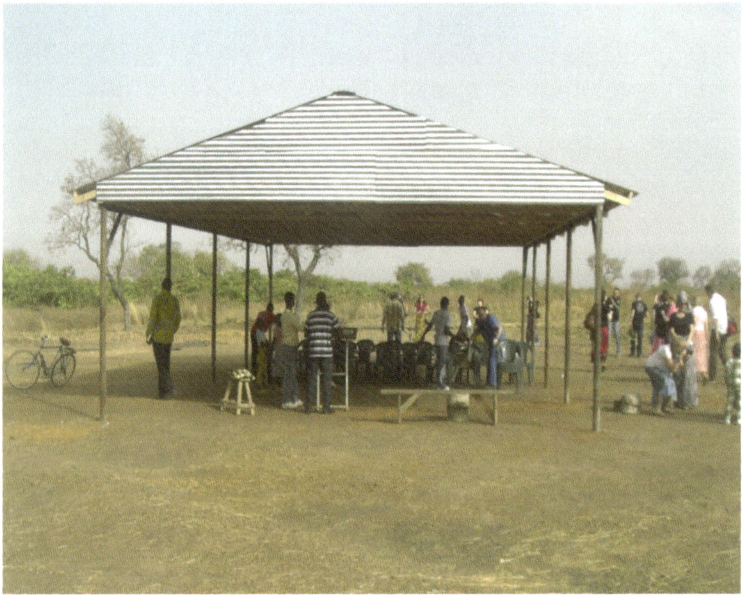

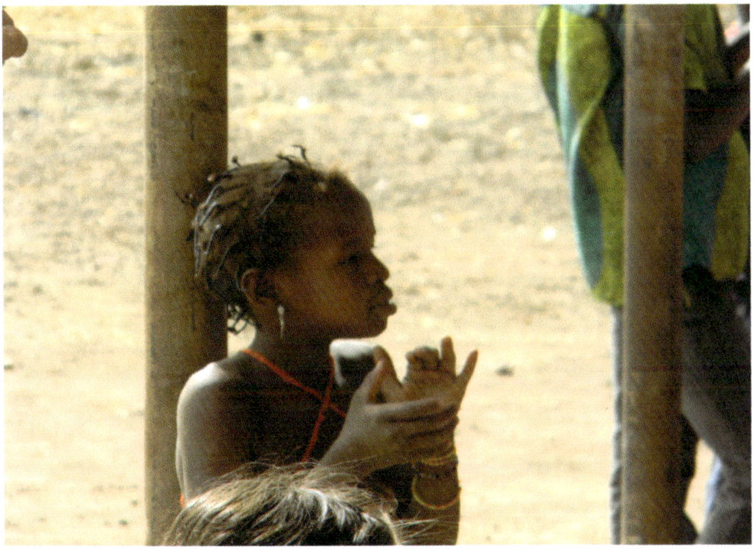

A Young Church Goer

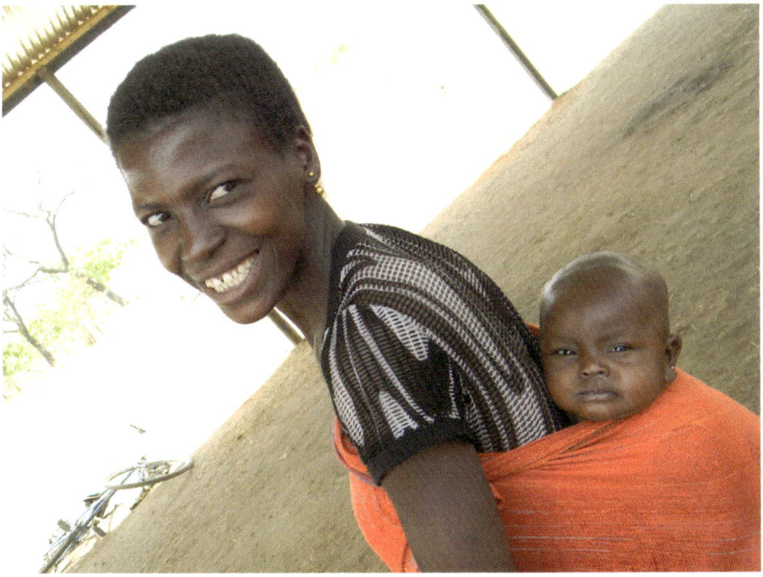

One Of Many Who Thirst

Church began at 9:15 a.m. Someone called to start the praise and worship part of the services. Approximately 25 Africans went to the front of the church and began to chant something to the beat of a drum. They were also clapping their hands. This went on for quite some time and of course, no one in our group understood what they were singing. After the singing stopped, Some´ said the first song was "Holy, Holy is He" and the second song was "Jesus is the Way."

A woman started to lead the next song. It was a lively, spirited song and she started to dance. A young girl accompanied her by slightly tossing a basket in the air that had shells or rocks attached to the edge of the basket. It made a sound like a maraca and added much to the song.

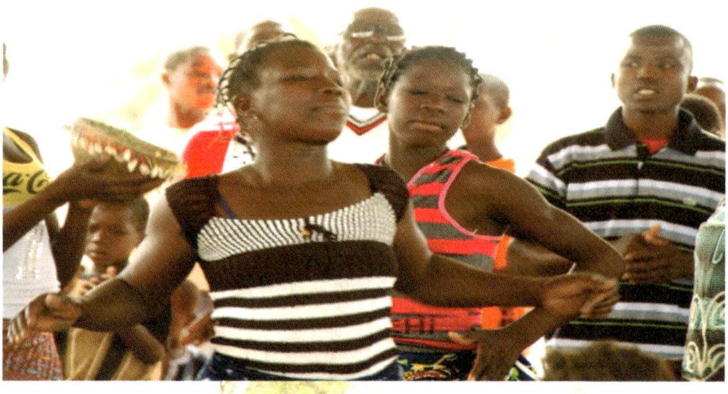

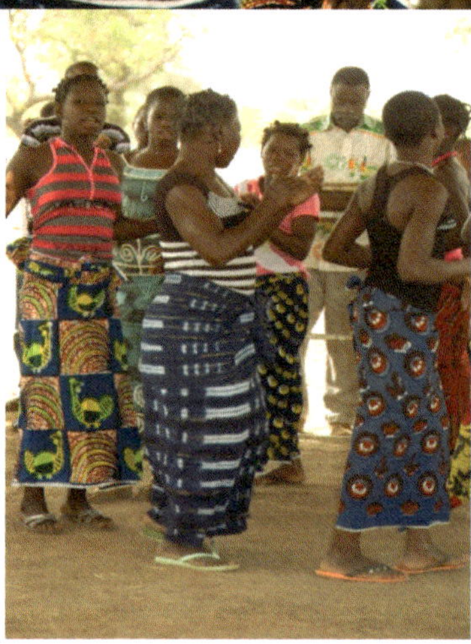

The song was a song with an echo. The leader would sing and the rest of the congregation echoed her words. Then things became exciting. The music intensified and the volume escalated. The leader then started to jump up and down and two other young girls joined her. Then the grand finale—the leader and the girls did the Lobi dance. They really had some moves going on! But, we enjoyed their worship services.

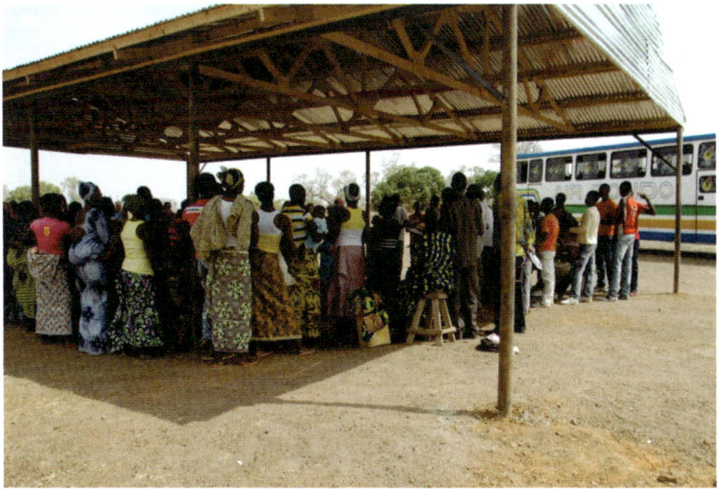

Praising The Lord

Some´ said that the Africans wanted our group to sing to them. We all stood and sang, "I'll Fly Away" and "Amazing Grace." I stood at the back of the group because I had been writing and was late getting with the group. As we sang, I noticed tears were flowing down the cheeks of several in our crowd. I lost it too when we sung, "When we've been there ten thousand years, bright shining as the sun; We've no less days to sing his praise, than when we've first begun." I couldn't finish the song. I was staring at the Africans and thought that the same God who loved us (me) also loved each and every one of them; that He had blessed us abundantly and He had blessed them the same. It may not appear that way because I think that sometimes being blessed is defined as ownership of wealth, health, possessions, successes, accomplishments, and does not consider the eternal blessings of being a child of the King. I felt the Africans might look more at the eternal because they had nothing else to consider. So who was really blessed and possibly more appreciative of what God had done for them?

The next topic on the agenda was for the young to lead in song and dance. The teenage girls danced in a circle while smaller children danced on the side. It was obvious one little boy around 3 years of age needed to go to the bathroom as he danced. I do not think he was doing the Lobi dance but the "happy dance"—a dance parents have seen during the process of toilet training their children.

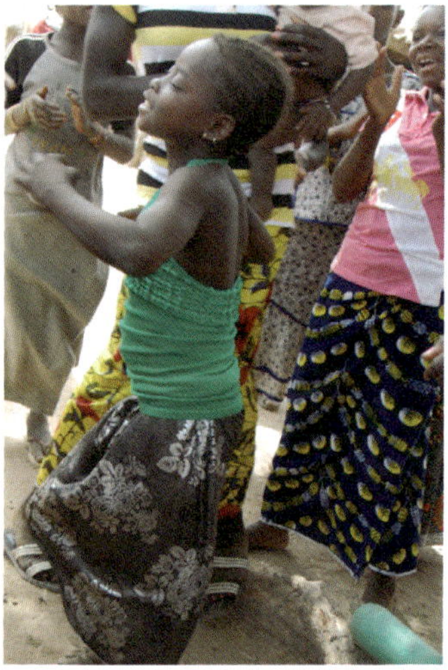

Young Girl Enjoying Worship

Church started. The pastor began preaching while Some´ interpreted. To sum-up his message: The pastor said, "Christians should give because they want to give and not because they are forced. What God gives us, He wants it to be used for His glory." He also said that they would like to build a new church by enclosing the framed structure with brick. He asked for us to pray that God gives them the things they will need to build. Then Some´ asked if anyone from our group wanted to speak. The pastor from a church in Oklahoma stood and began to speak. He told the African group that God would make a way for their needs to be met. Then we were instructed to gather around the exterior of the church, hold hands and pray that God would continue to bless the work that was yet to be done. This gathering of the saints was an emotional experience for many.

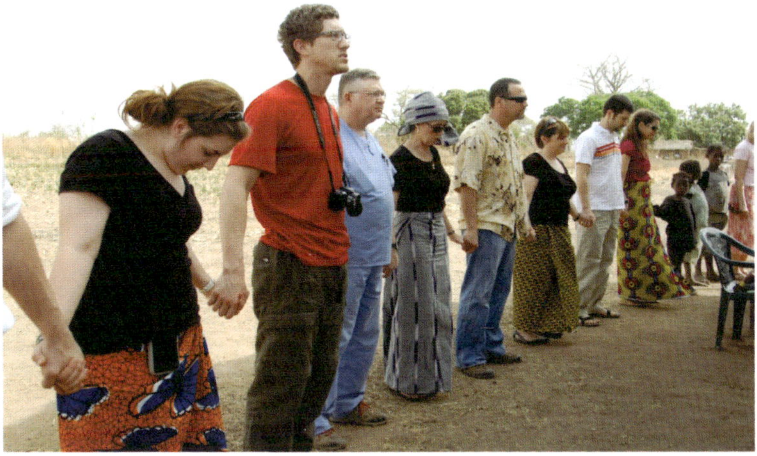

Gathering For Prayer

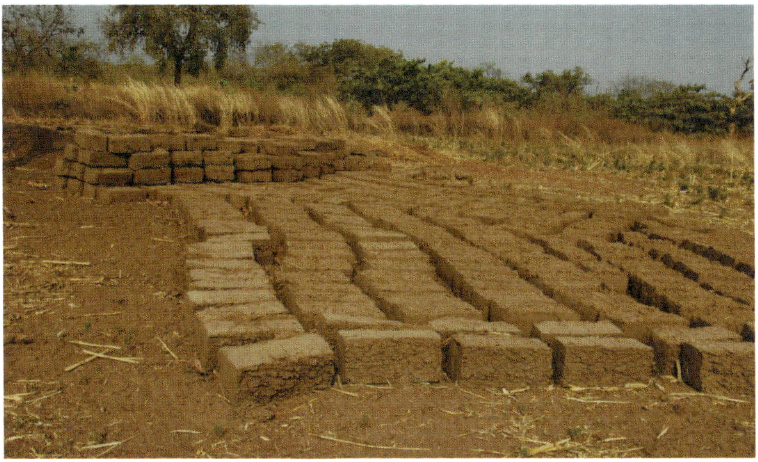

Mud Bricks Needed To Complete Building The Church.

We sat back down and the church took an offering. Everyone stood and chanted and clapped their hands. Two girls walked around carrying a wooden box and collected money. There were about six little kids sitting behind my husband, Dale and me. They were dirty unlike the other children. Dale said you could tell the children whose parents were not Christian by their cleanliness. I was glad they attended the church services because they heard preaching in their own language. What they heard will not return void. God said so.

The preaching began again. The pastor basically talked about the voice from heaven is God and we should listen to Him because He sent a deliverer for us so that we might go to heaven. He came to help us. The pastor spoke in French. Some´ interpreted in English and then in Lobi so that another interpreter could speak to his people.

There was a time for testimony after the preaching. Several from our group thanked the pastor for inviting us to the services. The preacher then asked if anyone wanted to be a believer that day. Four adult women and a young man went forward. They wanted prayer so that they might know what to do. Some wore colorful bands on their arms that indicated they worshipped the fetish gods. Jim from our group came forward and led in prayer over the congregation. After the prayer, the young man wanted to be saved! Dale was thrilled to be the one who led him to the Lord. The chief of the village and his brother witnessed this transformation. It was good for them to see because they accepted Christ as Savior just a few months earlier. This would help strengthen their faith and encourage them to reach others in the village.

We prayed once again before the dismissal song was sung. The drums began. It was another lively, spirited song. I noticed that one little boy standing on the side was a real ham. He was so cute as he danced and smiled broadly. The song was quite long. When it was over, Some´ said the name of the song was, “Jesus is coming back soon!”

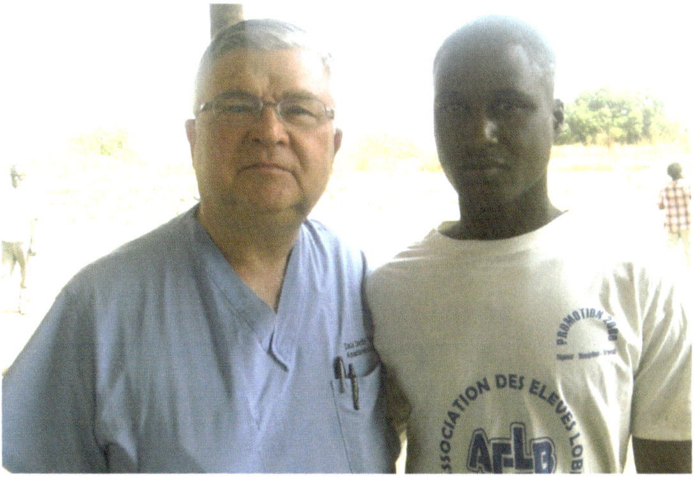

Dale With New Convert

Those words, "Jesus is coming back soon" touched my heart. Not only were the words exciting to think about but the words also served as a warning—a warning that supports Scripture. The fields for harvesting (souls) are truly great but the laborers are few. We should pray to the Lord of the harvest that He would send forth laborers into His harvest. (Luke 10:2) Therefore, we believers have a great job to do. We have been commissioned to take the Good News into all nations—teaching them to observe all the things God commanded and baptize them in the Name of the Father, Son and the Holy Spirit. (Matt 28: 19 – 20) It is our responsibility to spread the Good News to all people and we must do so quickly because time is short and Jesus is truly coming back again very soon.

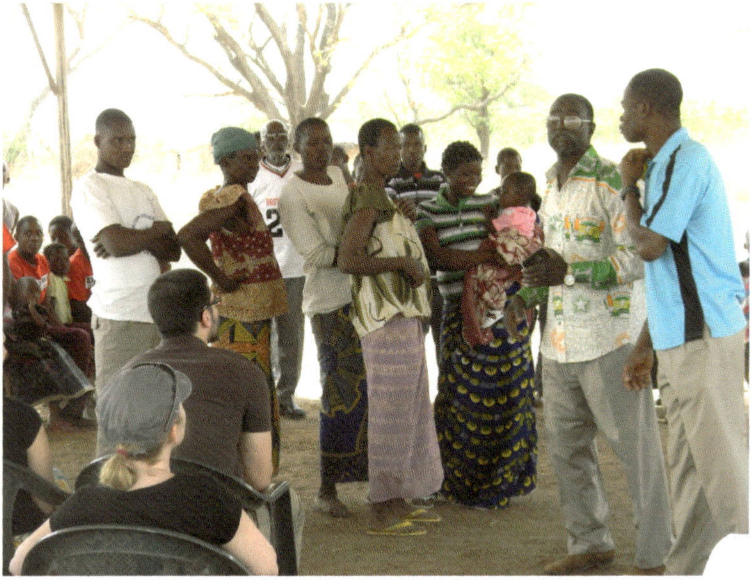

Fetish Worshippers Requesting Prayer To Believe

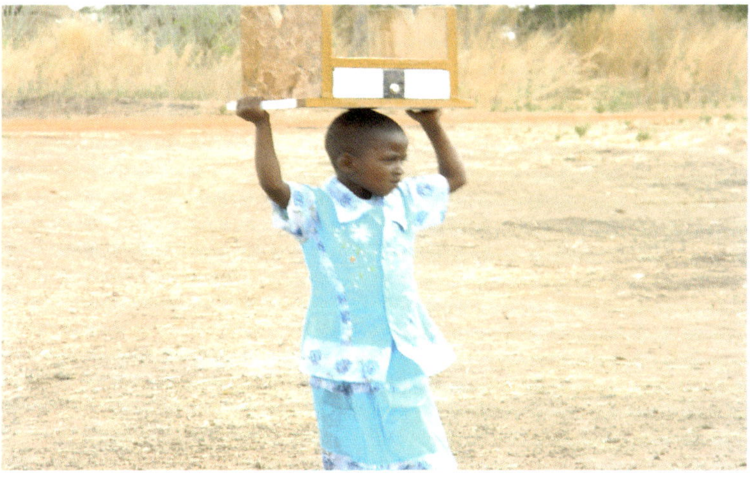

Carrying A Table To Church

THE VILLAGE OF THE LADY IN PINK

The women who were dressed in Lobi garb changed clothes on the bus after church services. Walking around in the village would be much easier in comfortable clothing.

The village was about the average size for African villages. There were approximately 20 huts and all basically made the same—with mud bricks. The mud consisted of dirt and hog dung. Hog dung is used because straw is already in the excrement and straw is needed for the consistency of the mud to make bricks. The roofs on the huts are thatched and are not very strong. Several roofs on the huts had fallen through and needed replaced. Some of the buildings had flat roofs. Dale and I actually climbed to the top and stood on the roof of one such hut. Villagers used the flat roofs of their huts to dry vegetables.

Hogs roamed free everywhere. They went in and out of the huts with ease and without fear. Chickens roamed around as well. African chickens are rather skinny as are the hogs. Not very much to eat would be my guess. There were also goats roaming about. It was like a little farm within the village proper.

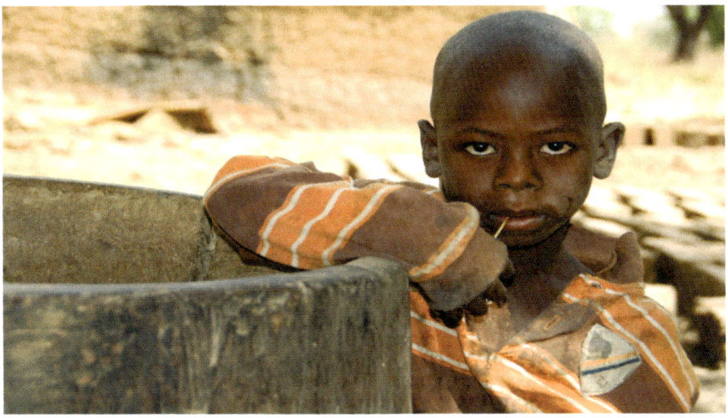

Eyes Of Interest And Fear

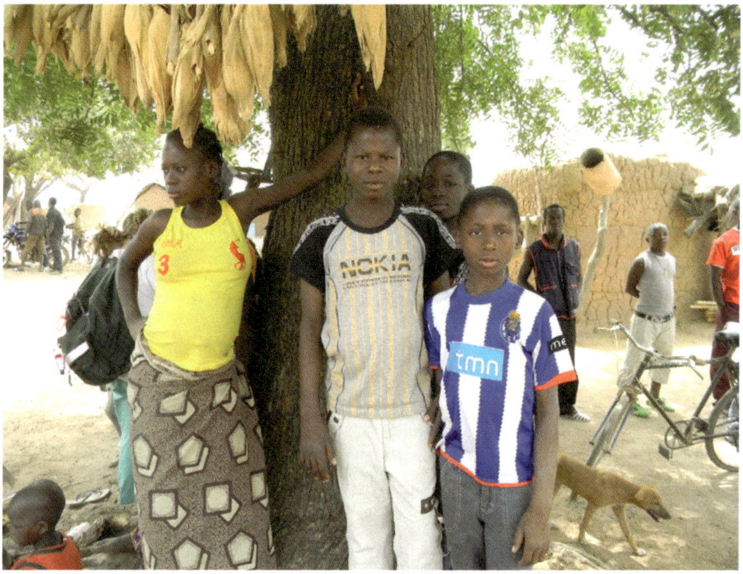

Village Kids

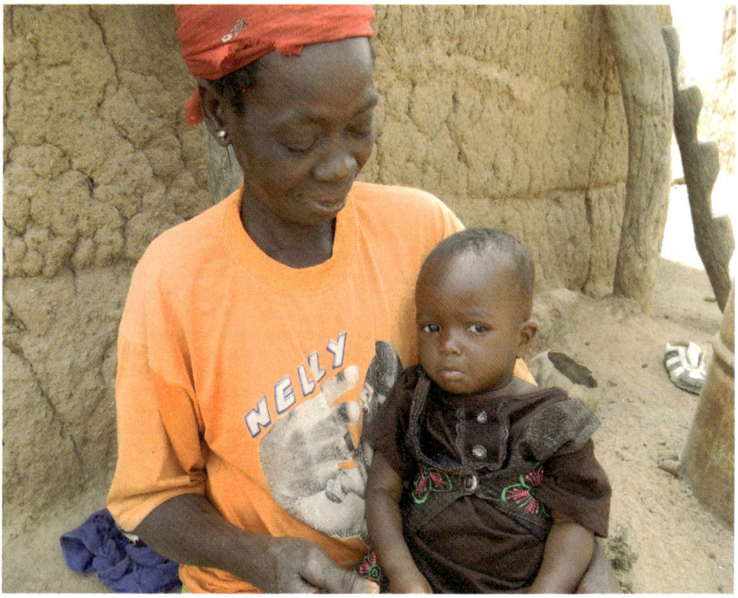

Waiting For Wound Treatment

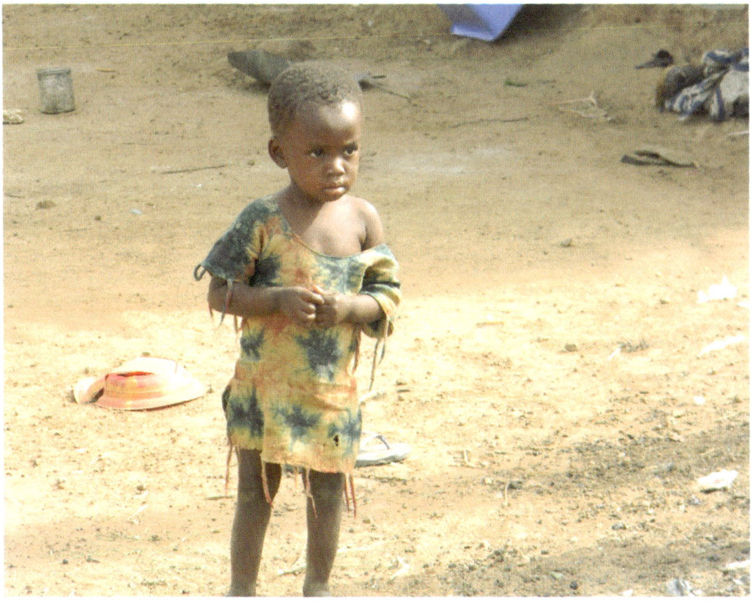

A Lad With A Questioning Look

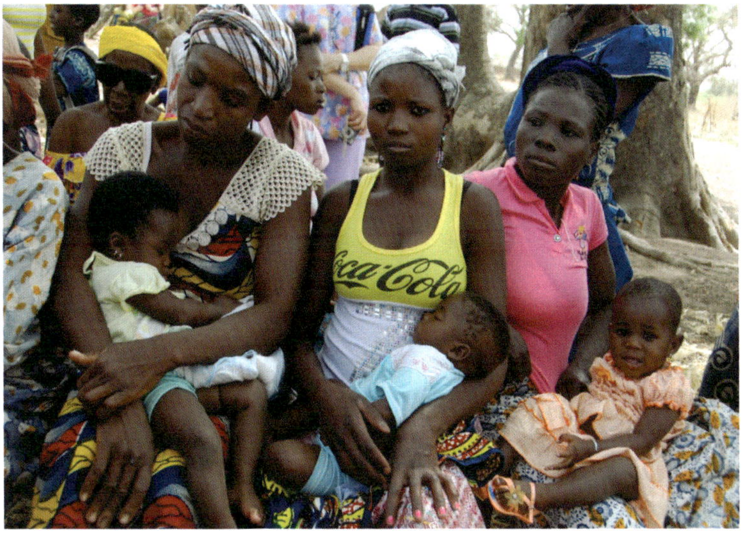

Mothers Welcome The Medical Personnel

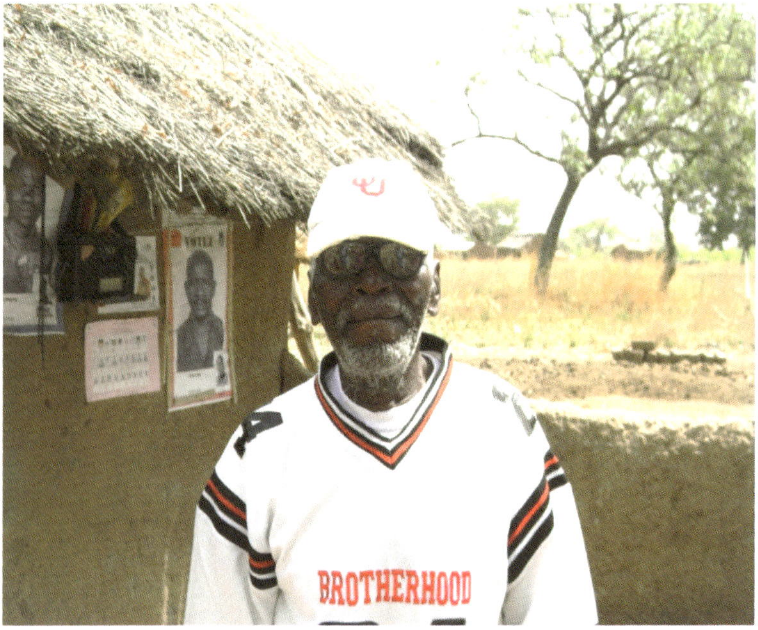

The Chief Of The Village And His Hut

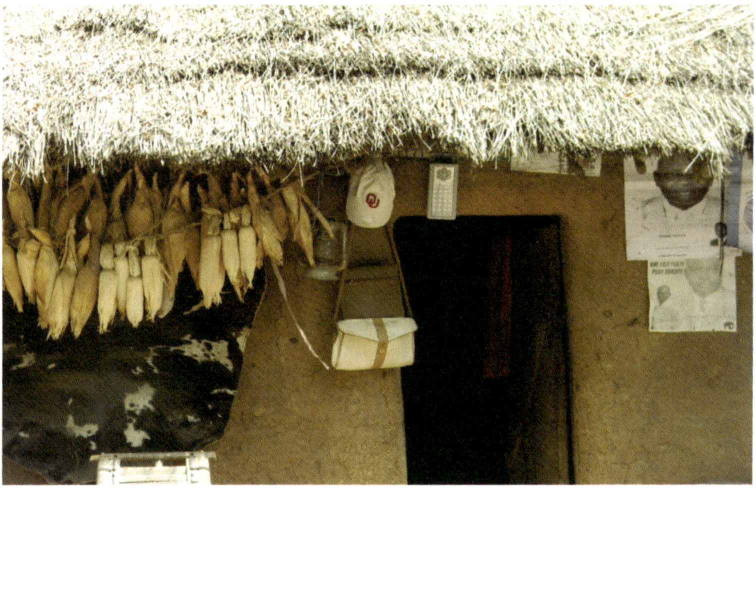

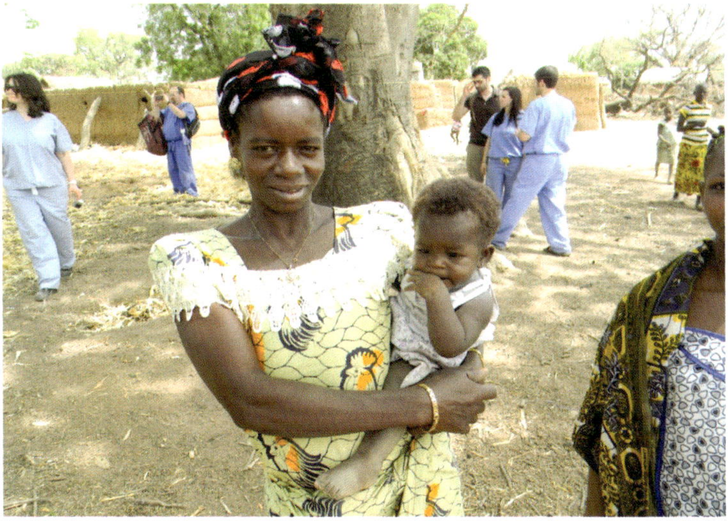

Mother And Child From The Village

Children were well behaved. They played as all children do and seemed to play well with others. There was a game they played that was similar to backgammon. They dug approximately 6 small holes in the dirt and filled these holes with small black pebbles. I did not know how the game was actually played but several of these games could be found dug-out in the dirt outside the family hut.

The men did not seem to have a great deal to do as far as I could tell. They sat around under the shade tree and chatted. This particular village was mostly Christian and perhaps the men were obeying God by resting on the Sabbath. Some´ said that very few Muslims lived in this area. Most lived in the surrounding villages but they do not give the Christians any trouble. Some´ also said that the Muslims that lived in this area do not really know why they were Muslim. Being Muslim was more of a family tradition. I mentioned to Some´ that it would appear that this group would be easy to reach with the Gospel since they do not know who they are spiritually or why they are Muslim. I mentioned that we could tell them what they could become with Christ. He agreed and said, "That is why we are here."

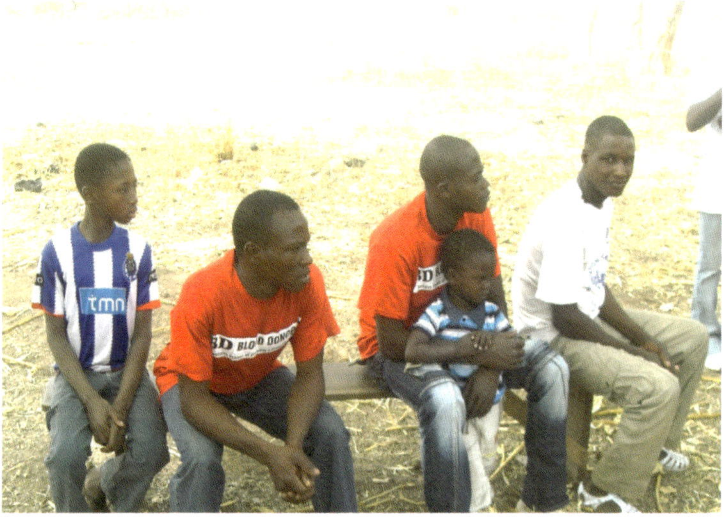

Men And Boys In The Village

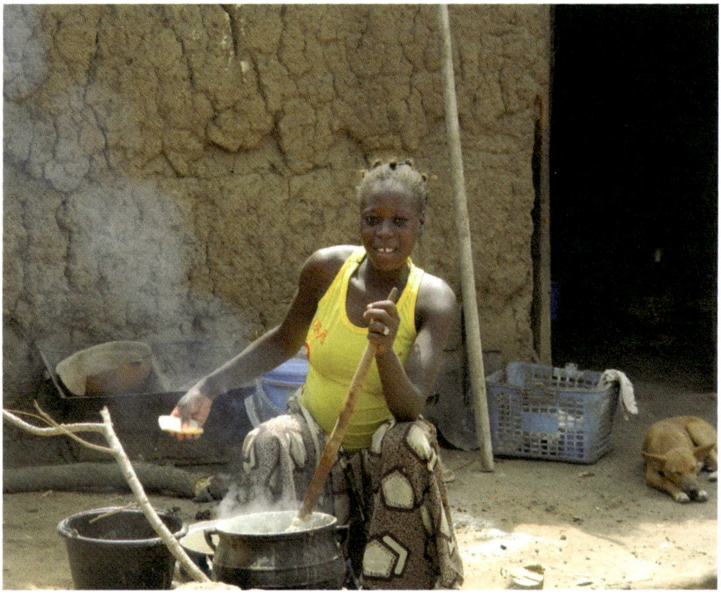

Woman Intent In Her Chores

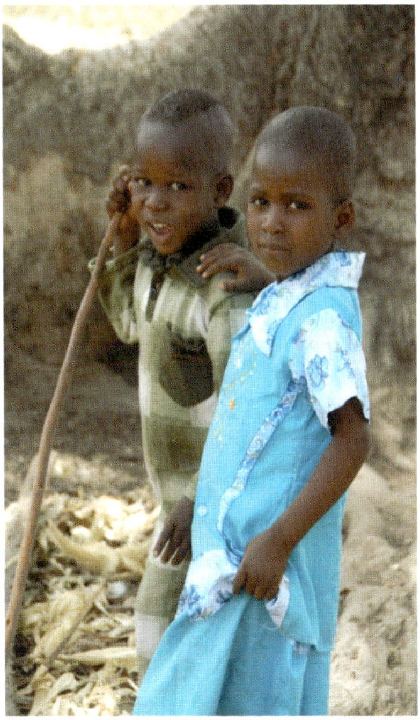

Children Of The Village

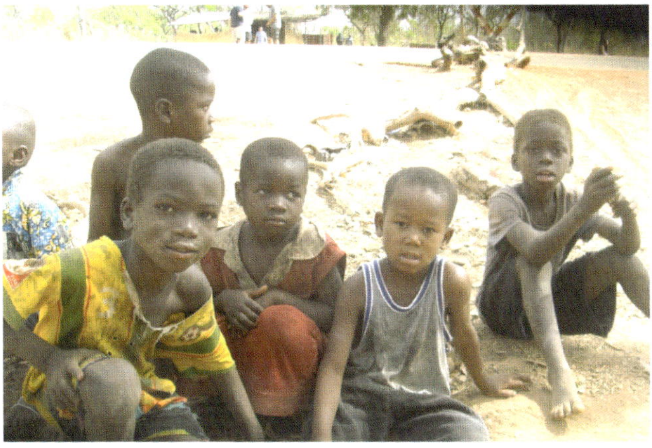

Dr. John was with our group. He gave first aid to some of the villagers with scrapes and scratches. There were so many children with foot sores and wounds—all potentially dangerous for getting infected and causing extreme problems. One lady Dr. John treated had attended church services earlier. I remembered her because of the pink outfit she wore but also because she did not look like she felt well. Dr. John said the woman had ovarian cancer and was in the end stages of the disease. She was in a great deal of pain so he gave her the pain medication he had. Her prognosis was extremely poor and she would probably die within the next 6 months. The only thing good about the prognosis was she was a believer and she would be going to heaven to be with the Lord. To be absent from the body is to be present with the Lord.

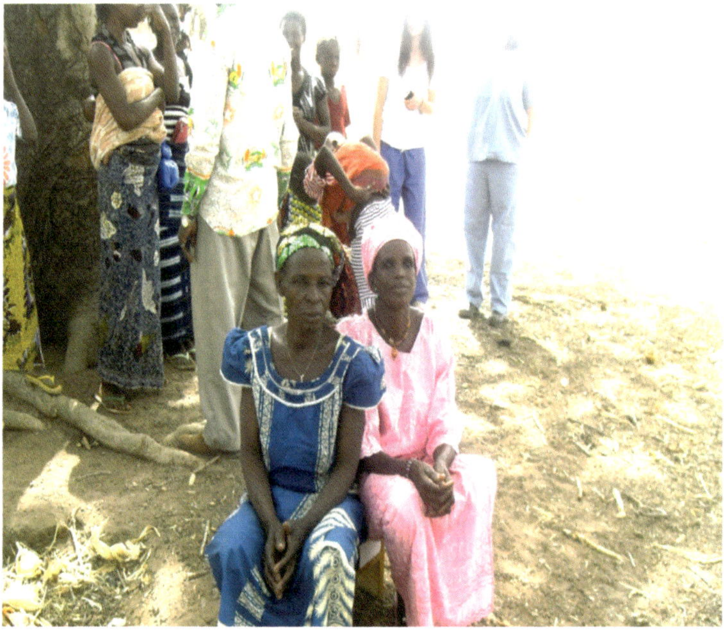

The Lady In Pink And A Friend

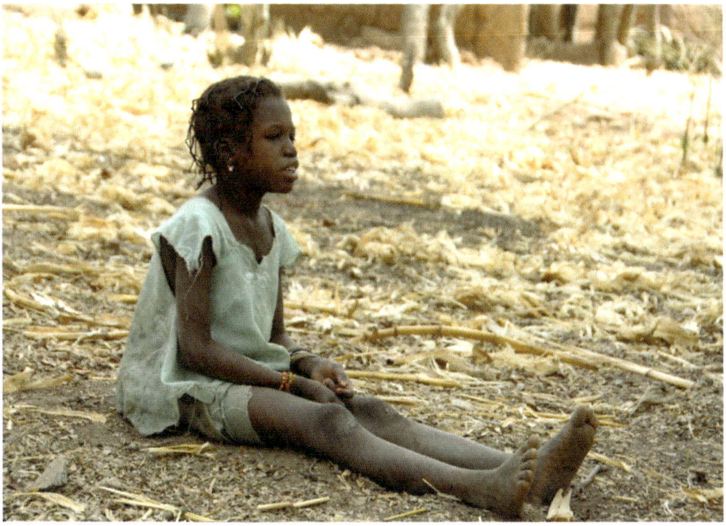

**Young Girl Curiously Watching
The American Strangers**

Most of the villagers wandered in under the shade tree to observe the first aid being given and perhaps just because of their curiosity. It reminded me of the masses who came to see and hear Jesus speak—curious perhaps but also in great need. Some of the villagers who gathered around were looking for healing but not realizing that real healing could only be found in Jesus Christ. Christ could give them hope that healed and restored lives and was lasting unlike the band-aid given with our first aid.

Russ and Tina were a couple from the Oklahoma City area that had made numerous trips to Africa with the group. Russ started to talk with me about the church we attended earlier in the day. Russ had been responsible to help raise money for the church structure. He told me that the church now sat in an old cornfield. He asked me if I knew the movie, Field of Dreams and the famous saying, "Build it and they will come?" Russ said that was exactly what they did. They built it (the church) and the villagers came and were now going to church. Russ also said that he dedicated his part of the church in memory of his father, Wayman. Tina mentioned that his death made it financially possible for them to make the trip this year. She was sad that Wayman had died but was grateful she and Russ were able to go to Africa. I was reminded that even something as bad and painful as the death of a loved one, God could work it out for our good to those who loved Him and had been called according to His purpose.

The young girls in the village provided some entertainment by dancing in the town square. Some of the dances resembled hardcore aerobic exercises. It made me hurt to watch! They were having fun singing and dancing. One very tall young girl who looked to be about 15 years old got in on the action. She was very pretty and had a small baby tied to her back. I assumed the baby was her child. I thought to myself what a sad lot for young woman having so many children and the inability to adequately care for them, and the work involved caring for their needs without modern conveniences. I was careful not to get too caught up in their situation because like everyone had said, "It was all they knew."

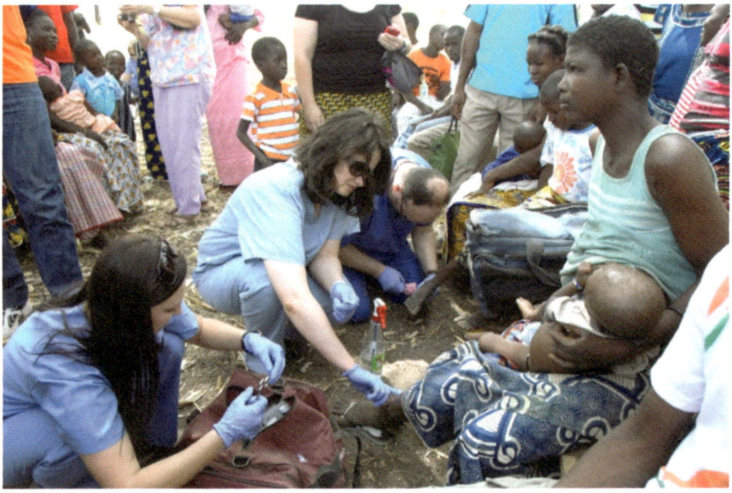

The Medical Team At Work

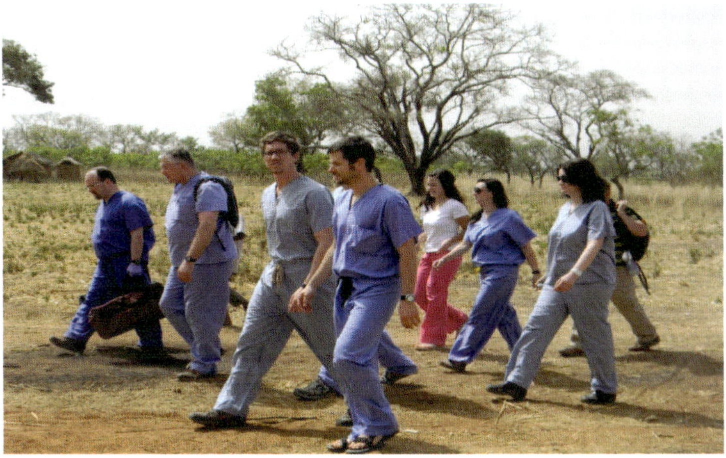

It was time to leave the village and board the bus for Camp Doropo. As we were pulling out, the entire village had gathered and was standing underneath the church structure. They were waving and saying good-bye in Lobi. It was a sight to behold—happy smiling faces, not necessarily because we were there, but because they knew the risen Savior, the benefits of the Cross—and were happy in the Lord.

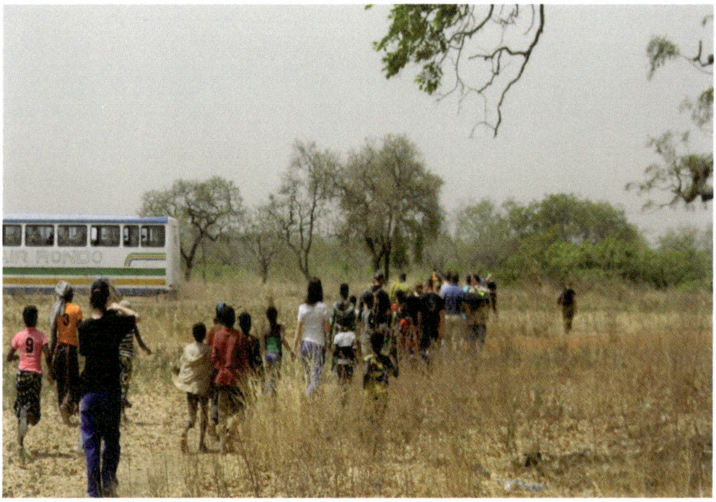

Escorting The Team Back To The Bus

The drive back to camp was hot and we were very thirsty. Once in our tent, Dale and I rested like we usually do on Sunday. I wrote in my journal of my experiences of the day as Dale tried to nap. It had been a wonderful Sabbath Day and my soul rejoiced.

Bless the Lord, O my soul; and all that is within me, bless His Holy Name. (Ps 103:1)

VALENTINE'S DAY—LOVE EXTENDED BY GOD

The wound care team had boarded the van around 9:00 a.m. to go into the villages to preach the Good News and care for the wounded. This was a real first for me spending Valentine's Day in 90 degree temperatures, dodging malaria carrying mosquitoes, and being deprived of even a morsel of sweet, delicious, chocolate—anywhere! But, I loved it.

The village we first visited was once named Colongo. When the old chief of the village, Dognesse, was dying, he appointed a new chief, a man named Binfie. A new appointed chief would sometime rename the village after themselves but Binfie did not want to do so. Binfie renamed the village Dogbi in order to honor chief Dognesse. Binfie had three sons: Tchodifitae, Filaiminko, and Filpite. Filpite was now the new chief. He did not want to change the name of the village either but wanted to add to the village name. The name of the village became Dogbi Binfie.

There was a mix in the religions practiced in this village. Some villagers were Christian and others practiced the fetish religion. The village was a large village and I asked perhaps one of the dumbest questions ever. I asked the chief how large was his village. He acted as if I had asked him for his social security card or something. He looked bewildered. I then realized that no records of any kind are kept and people have no real concept of time, numbers, etc. However, he did respond and stated the village was large—very large.

The preacher, Devoria, asked the chief for permission to bring the Good News and then bring healing to their wounds. Devoria received permission from the chief and began to preach. He seemed to hold the attention of the villagers well. Several men who were listening interrupted the preacher. One said that it was difficult to accept God and would need to talk to other villagers later about whether to do this or not.

The preacher stopped and wanted to pray for the man and he did but the man remained resistant and did not change his mind.

Two women came over to shake our hands. I asked Eli, our interpreter for the day, to ask them if they were Christian. They told him that they were and went to the Baptist Church at a different location. The two women wanted someone from the team to pull a couple of their teeth. Thankfully, we were unable to oblige this request because we did not have any pliers. Seriously!

The preacher began to preach once again. The women were praying for the preacher and his message. When the preacher stopped, we circled with the people to pray. When we were finished, the pastor asked if anyone wanted to receive Christ as Savior. Five adult men responded and were saved! The preacher wrote their names down in a ledger so that he could make a follow-up visit later.

The team began with the wound care. We saw the usual foot injuries but they were nothing compared to their other medical needs we were unable to treat. Toothbrushes were also handed out and the children really liked them. We gathered up our equipment, said good-bye to the villagers, and left to go to the next village.

Village Number Two

The name of the next village was Tchartchari. The team got out of the van and walked a short distance to the village. Several adults led us to the shade tree in the center of the village. One young man went to get the chief. In the meantime, women and children gathered close.

The chief came to meet and welcome us. His name was Chief Kambou Gborobi. Eli, our Lobi interpreter, asked if we could come and give them the Good News and encouragement. He agreed for us to do so and then said we come every year and he was very grateful.

Pastor Devoria began to preach. (Pastor Devoria was from the Doropo Church.) There were approximately 30 people present not counting the children. The preacher gave a short message but asked at the end if anyone wanted to accept Christ as Savior. He then said if they did, they were to repeat after him the sinner's prayer. Many adults and children repeated the prayer led by the preacher. The pastor wrote down the names of those who were saved that day and there were five. He would make follow-up visits later.

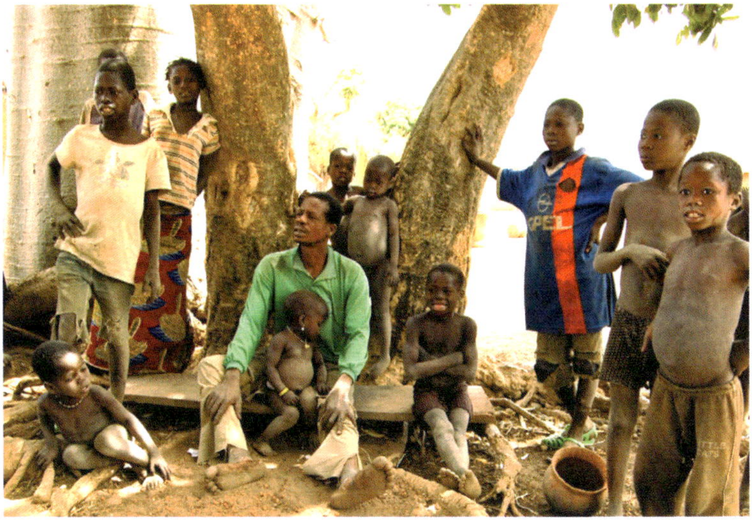

Chief Listens To The Good News

I asked Eli if the chief was a Christian. Eli spoke to him in Lobi and the chief said that he believed there was a God and talked to God every day. I asked Eli if the chief believed there was a God or if he believed in God and had a personal relationship with Him. The chief said that he had asked Jesus in his heart and knew God. I was happy to hear that.

Wound care began and ended quickly. Same scenario with the injuries of scrapes, abrasions, and cuts. There were just a few who needed to have their wounds dressed and there were no serious problems noted. We packed up and started our walk back to the van. As we were leaving I told the children that God loved them. Eli said for me to tell the children this in the Lobi language. Easy for him, I thought but he quickly taught me that Tangba Nafer (spelling may not be correct) was Lobi for Jesus loves you. I made many attempts to tell them Tangba Nafer. The children all smiled, possibly because I had botched the language so badly, and we waved good-bye.

We left the village and ventured down the road for a mile or so, pulled over to the side, and ate our lunch. Protein bars and Gatorade can be good in a pinch but a Snickers bar would have been better at least for Valentine's Day.

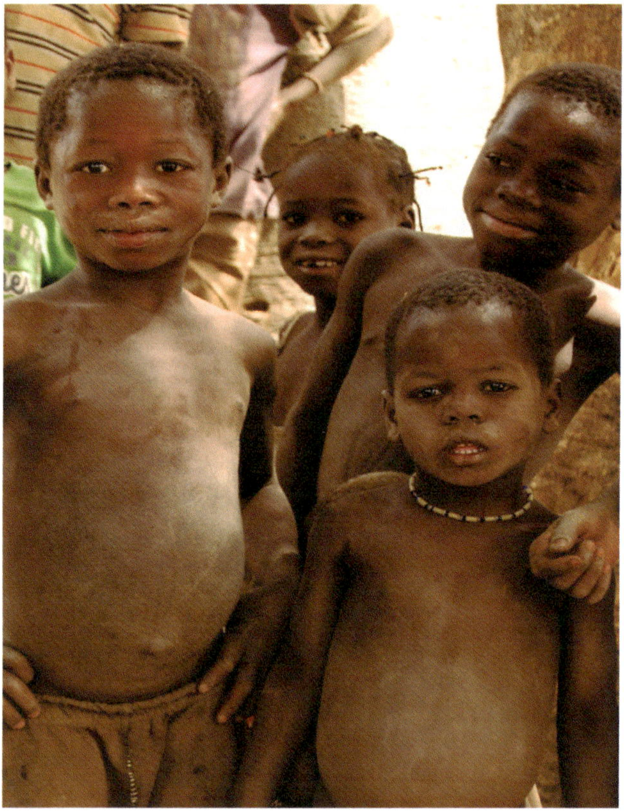

They Came, They Saw, And Some Believed.

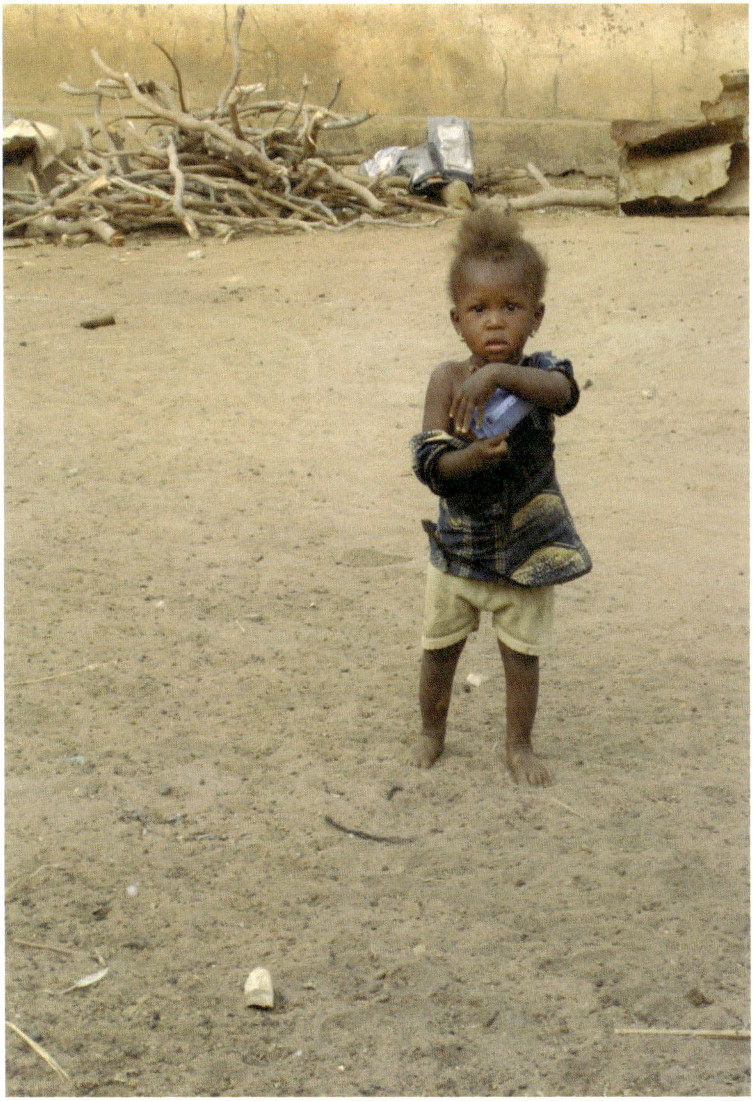

Is There Hope?

Village Number Three and the Blind Man

The name of the village was Biguinadoua. It sat a short distance off the road but the walk was easy. The village appeared to be a Christian village at first glance. The women were very friendly and greeted us and shook our hands. There seemed to be some community pride in the village in that the dirt looked swept outside their huts and there was no trash anywhere. The village looked clean as the conditions allowed. But there were signs that the fetish religion was also practiced. Dried gourds were hanging from sticks that were standing upright in the fields and by several huts.

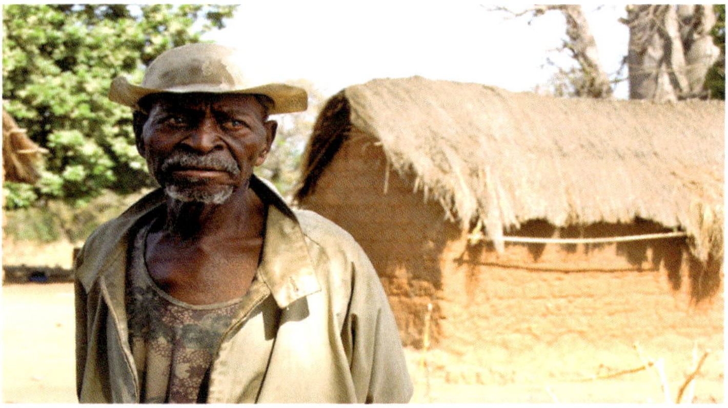

The Village Chief

We assembled under a large tree a few yards from the huts. Approximately 60 people gathered around. Several young children found chairs for the group to sit on. The chairs had been made by the villagers and were quite comfortable. They were made with sticks or small limbs and woven together. The chief was summoned and he came to meet us a few minutes later. He gave permission for us to bring the Good News and give wound care.

With this village, Pastor Devoria used a book entitled, “Good News” as his means for sharing the Gospel. He quickly went through the book while showing them the illustrations. I noticed a young adult male standing almost behind the shade tree and definitely away from the group. I could tell he was blind but was listening to what the preacher had to say. I also saw a young man crawling on his legs to get closer to the preaching. People with physical handicaps are considered outcasts. Other villagers have nothing to do with them. They are often ridiculed and mistreated by people within their village.

The preacher saw the blind man and when he concluded his message, he prayed a prayer for those who did not know Christ to accept Him that day. Then the preacher asked for special prayer for the blind man and had the blind man to come closer to stand near him. Then they began to pray and so did our group. Thirteen people accepted Christ as Savior while standing under the shade tree. They heard the Good News for the first time and their eyes were opened to God's truths. However, the icing on the cupcake was—the blind man had also been saved.

I asked Eli to find out if the blind man was blind at birth. He asked and said that he went blind a short time after birth. The blind man was smiling and seemed extremely happy. In fact, I never saw him not smile from the time of his salvation until we left the village.

Wound care was pretty much the same as in the other villages. I stood back and observed while the team members administered care. I wanted to write but my writing was soon interrupted when two women came to me holding their small children. With Eli interpreting, one woman said her little girl was about 3 years old and could not walk. I looked at the child. She was tiny for her age and I noticed her lower extremities were not as developed as her upper body. I asked the mother if the child could stand. She tried to stand the little girl on the ground but she screamed as if in pain. The mother held her once again.

The situation with the other child was the same. I concluded that the two little girls had either been stricken with polio at one point, or meningitis, or possibly some other neurological problem. I told them there was nothing we could do. I felt bad in that there was nothing we could do and unless by a miracle, these little girls would grow up and be outcasts in the village because they would not be able to walk.

During wound care, a mother appeared holding a young boy approximately 5 years old. He was noticeably sick. He was lethargic, feverish, and possibly septic. She laid him on her lap and showed us his problem. He had a 3-inch gash in the left inguinal area and it was so deep the tendons or possibly the fascia were visible. (It was difficult to determine from where I was standing.) I felt he was definitely septic. I told Bob that the boy needed to go to the hospital ASAP. His wound needed immediate attention, possibly an I & D, (incision and drainage) and placed on IV antibiotics. Tina wrote a note and gave to the mother to give the triage nurse at the hospital that we had sent the child in for treatment. The mother found a villager that gave her and the child a ride to town on the moped.

Later I discovered that the nurse at the hospital had seen the child and the mother had been instructed to bring the boy back the first thing in the morning for treatment. To my knowledge neither the mother nor the patient returned the next day. Unless the child was later treated, he would most surely die.

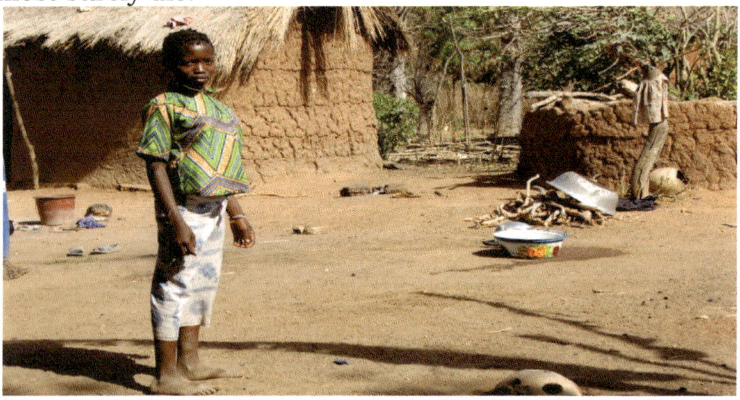

An Interested Follower

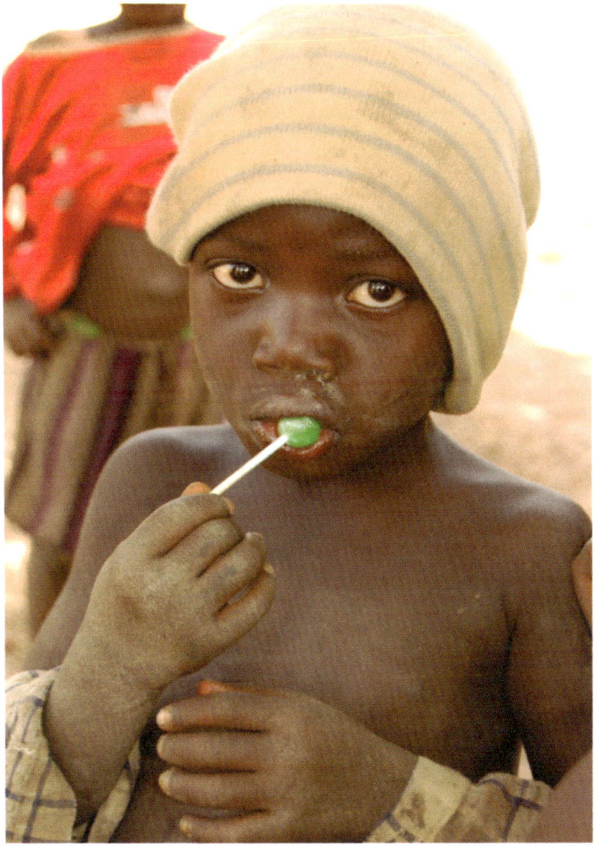

Eyes That Search

Tina had a bag of bon-bons (candy suckers) she wanted to give to the children. Amazingly, the adults wanted the treats as well. Eli called the group to order and had the children and adults to form a line to receive the candy. Tina stood on one side of the line and I on the other side. As the children and adults walked passed us, Tina gave them the candy and I told them that Jesus loved them—Tangba Nafer.

It was time to leave the village and return to camp. We were walking back to the van and I noticed the blind man was following us on the path. He had a stick to aid his footing and was walking cautiously. He was smiling happily. My heart broke for this young man. If things were not bad enough just living in squalor, he had to do it being blind! I felt the need to say something to him. I asked Eli to help translate. I told Eli to tell the blind man that when he opened his eyes in heaven, the first face he would see would be that of his Savior.

I was emotional as I spoke to the blind man. I remembered reading once about Fanny Crosby, the great hymn writer of all time. She was blinded as a newborn baby. She was asked during an interview during her later years if she had any regrets being blind all her life. Her response was, "No not really—because the first face I will see when I open my eyes in heaven will be that of my Savior."

What I experienced that day coupled with my knowledge of Fanny Crosby reminded me of the chorus to the song, "What A Day That Will Be" by Jim Hill:

What a day that will be; When my Jesus I shall see;
When I look upon His face; The One who saved me by his Grace;
When He takes me by my hand; And leads me to the Promised Land;
What a Day, Glorious Day that will be!

It can't get any better than that!

MEETING "KING AGRIPPA"

It was difficult to believe that this day would be the last field day the wound care team would make into the villages. The week passed so quickly. I had an incredible time going into the villages, talking with the people, assessing their needs, playing with the children, watching God work, and being reminded how important and urgent was our responsibility to tell others the Good News of Jesus Christ. I was excited about today as we ventured out into the uttermost parts of the world.

The name of the village we were to visit was Kakota. The van was parked several "blocks" from the actual village so our group had to walk the remaining distance. Before we started the trek to the village, the group wanted to look around at the small brick church that stood close by. This structure had been built the previous year by the construction team from our group. The building looked to be about a 15 X 20 foot structure. The interior was dirt and a distinct place had been prepared for the pastor to stand as he preached the message. It was marked-off by a layer of brick and the pastor would stand inside that area. There were also three windows and two open doors for ventilation. It was primitive but quite functional and a nice place for worship.

Pastor Abel was our pastor who went with the wound care team that morning. We walked to the village but we could not meet with the chief because he was in Doropo. We had to go to plan B and meet the next authority in line. While Pastor Abel attempted to make that connection with the next in line, the rest of the team walked around and viewed the countryside. We stood on a huge granite boulder that was partially exposed above the ground that served as a large flat plateau. We were able to overlook the village and the surrounding area. Several villagers were walking on the path surrounding their village unaware of our presence. We heard children laughing and watched them play in the tall grass of the fields. It was very hot standing on that boulder without any shade from the African sun.

Pastor Abel had been successful in his connections and we were allowed to go into the village and give the Good News and wound care. The village looked clean. The huts were tidy and the dirt outside their homes appeared swept. However, there were signs that some of the villagers worshiped the fetish gods. The signs of fetish worship can usually be seen in the center of the village as they were in this particular village. There were sticks or limbs standing in the dirt with a dried-out gourd attached at the top. A chicken had been killed and the blood sprinkled on the limb holding the gourd. Of interest, which ever the way a chicken fell after the throat had been cut, determined if it was a good sacrifice or not. If the chicken fell on its back, the fetish worshippers considered that to be a good sacrifice. If the chicken fell in any other direction, either to the front or to either side, it was not a good sacrifice. After the chicken died, the blood was sprinkled on the limb holding the gourd. It made no difference if the sacrifice was considered to be good or bad, the blood was still sprinkled. Then they would cook and eat the chicken. I can't imagine eating a chicken that was considered to be a bad sacrifice. It made no sense to me.

We followed a group of villagers to a large tree where chairs were brought for us to sit on. In this particular village I noticed the women were very chatty. In fact, they talked constantly to each other and tried to communicate with us. I also noticed that African women yell at their children as they disciplined. Perhaps that was why the children were well behaved.

The chief finally emerged from his hut. He was wearing a black cap. Several children followed him. He appeared to be very old. His name was Kambou Tihanie. His eyes for some reason fascinated me as I had been with other older villagers. His eyes were gentle and full of sights known only to him.

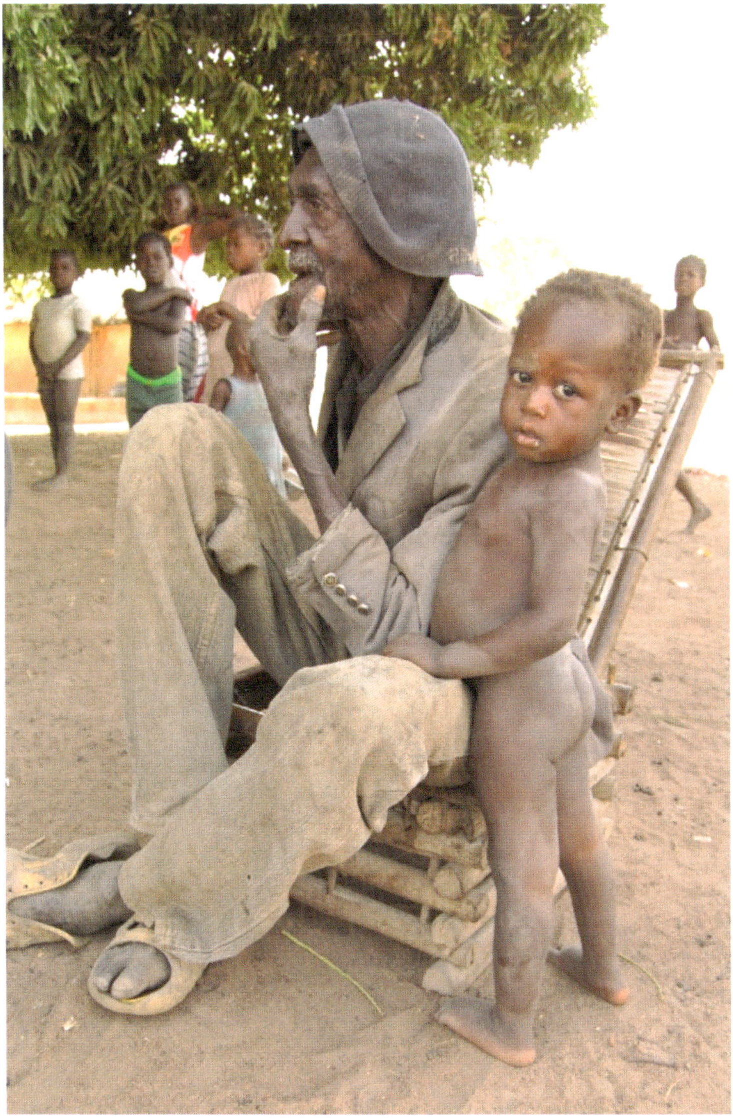

The Substitute Chief Of The Village, The Modern Day "King Agrippa"

Eli, our interpreter, sounded the bullhorn to get the attention of the villagers so they would be able to hear the Good News and receive healing for their wounds. Approximately 50 people came and gathered around the tree. Pastor Abel began preaching. He held their attention well. Then the pastor ended the message and Eli prayed a very long prayer. No one accepted Christ and became a believer.

Pastor Abel approached the chief and was talking to him as the wound care team began to dress the cuts and wounds of the villagers. I asked Eli what was exactly taking place between the chief and Pastor Abel. Eli said that the real chief to the village was in the hospital in Doropo and this substitute chief was the chief's brother. The substitute chief said that he had heard the Good News before but was not convinced to believe. He did not mind for the children to go to the church but he was not ready to make that decision. Pastor Abel asked the chief why he did not want to go to church or become a believer. The chief said that it is a personal decision and he wanted his children to convince him this was good. The chief said that his brother was a Christian and when he returned from the hospital he would ask him what to do. He said that accepting Christ should not be done because someone tells you to do so. Eli told me that the substitute chief's heart was very hard and resistant. Then the chief said, "I was almost convinced to believe your message but I will wait another day." Pastor Abel explained to him that we had no guarantee of tomorrow and that he could die that day. The chief said, "I am not ready. Maybe later but not today."

I could hardly believe my ears. I had heard the words of King Agrippa repeated by a modern day King Agrippa, the substitute chief of the village. My heart ached. He had been enlightened by the Word of God and realized that he should become a believer but wanted to wait until later. What a dangerous path to take especially when living in an area of the world where death comes easily. Life is just a vapor and tomorrow is not guaranteed. To die without Christ would be unthinkable.

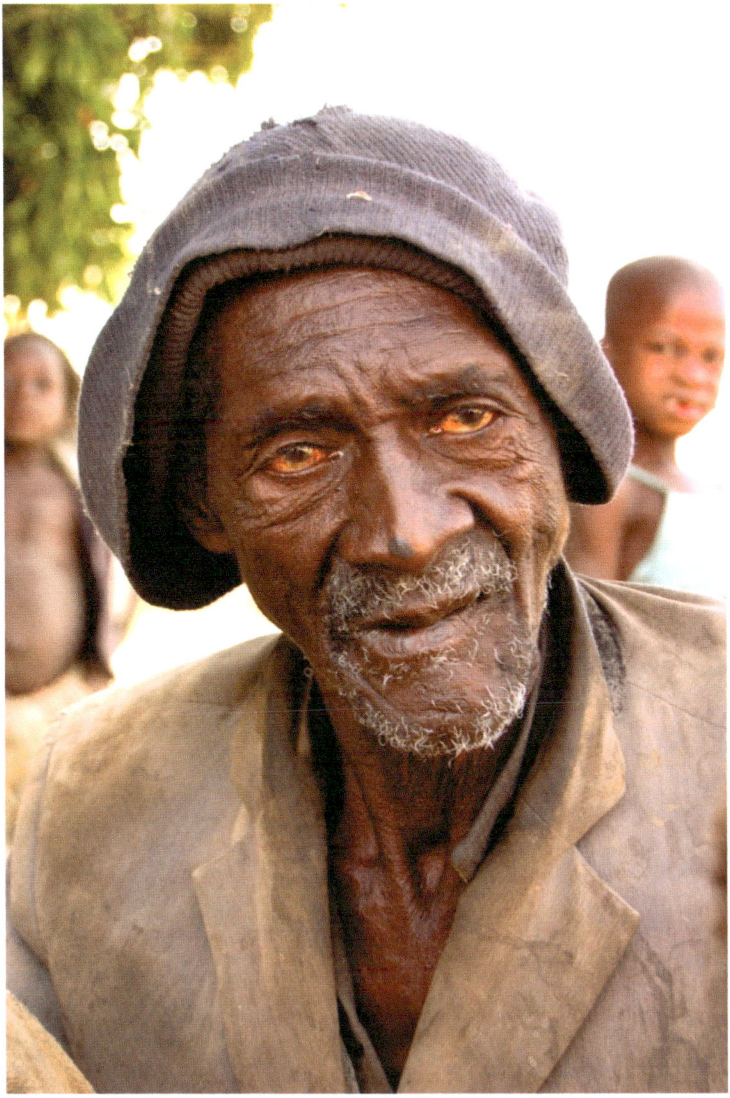

"King Agrippa"

Paul to King Agrippa: King Agrippa, do you believe the Prophets? I know that you believe. Then Agrippa said unto Paul, you almost persuaded me to become a Christian. Paul said, I would to God that not only you but also all who hear me this day, were both almost, and altogether such as I am except for these chains. (Acts 26:27-29)

Village Number Two

The name of the second village we visited was Tingo. In this particular village there were no chiefs but kings. The king's name was Ouattara Kouakou.

We got out of the van and walked a short distance to the village. The village was dirty and the people were not very friendly. Our interpreter, Eli, began speaking with several men standing nearby and told them why we were there and that he needed to speak to the king. They exchanged formalities and then they began to clap their hands for us. I thought that was a little strange but I went with the flow. Villagers from this village were referred to as members of the kingdom.

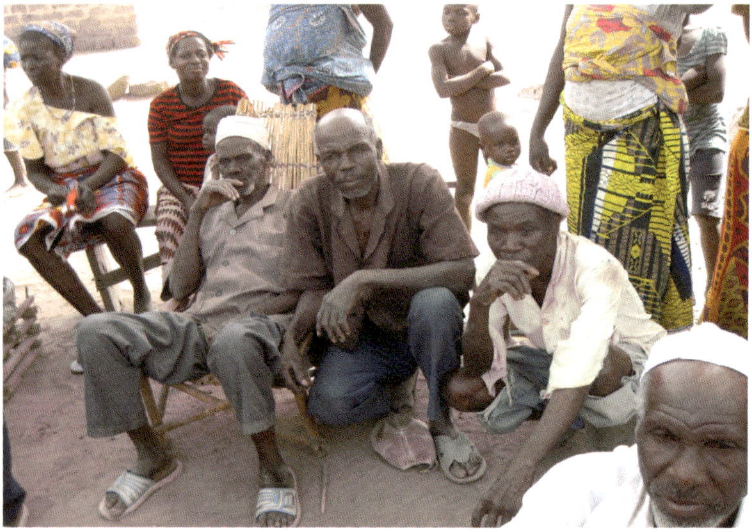

Note The Men With The Muslin Headwear

We walked toward the center of the town where many villagers sat under a huge baobab tree. The tree was absolutely enormous and provided a great deal of shade for the village. The children brought chairs for us to sit on and we did so. The king soon arrived on the scene. He wore a Muslim style hat, as did several of the village men. Eli approached the king and told him why we were there and he consented to let us teach the Good News and give wound care.

There were two different people groups in the village, Lobi and Koulango. The village was primarily Koulango. The king wanted Pastor Abel to preach in Lobi and not Koulango. Pastor Abel chose to speak in Koulango.

The pastor spoke to them directly and told the people of their need for Christ. He told them that they could not go to another life without Jesus Christ. He said that the fetishes offered other ways to another life but Jesus Christ was the only way to eternal life. He quoted John 14: 6. "Jesus said unto Him, I am the Way, the Truth, and the Life. No man comes unto the Father, but by me."

I was watching the crowd as Pastor Abel spoke. He held the attention of those present but the king appeared agitated. When Pastor Able finished his message, the king would not shake his or Eli's hand. He then left the group to go sit under a wood and straw structure where fetish gods are worshipped. No one accepted Christ that day.

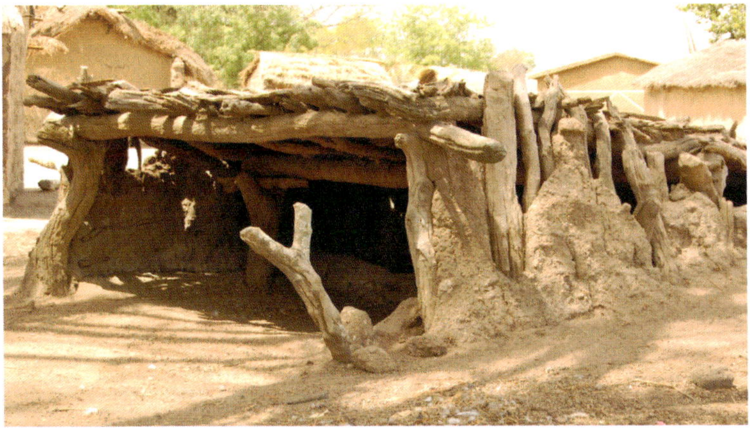

Place Where Fetish Gods Are Worshipped

Eli thought that the king was angry because Pastor Abel spoke in Koulango and not Lobi. He felt that the king did not want Koulango spoken because the villagers would be able to understand what Pastor Abel said. If the pastor spoke in Lobi, the villagers would not know what he had said. The king sounded like an evil king.

I observed and “felt” that this was a bad village that had been steeped in fetish religion for centuries. I had difficulty praying during the services. I felt the stronghold of Satan on this village. I sensed the evil presence. It was not a happy place to be and the people did not appear happy, even the children.

I concluded that the king was an evil king who temporarily lost control over his people. They were allowed to hear the Good News in their native language. They got what they wanted and he did not. I believed the Holy Spirit flexed His muscle and directed Pastor Abel to defy the king and speak to the people in Koulango.

It would be difficult for people to accept Christ who practiced fetish religions. How do we get people to believe in the one true God when they believe in so many other gods—fetish gods? How do we show them, convince them of the difference? How do we explain the Holy Spirit when they already believe in spirits and would consider Him as just another one? When they tell us that they believed in God, which god are they referring too?

Visiting this particular village made Ephesians 6:12 come alive. “For we wrestle not against flesh and blood but against principalities; against powers, against rulers of the darkness of this age; against spiritual hosts of wickedness in the heavenly places.”

We were disappointed that no one in the village was saved but were encouraged that many heard the Gospel preached in their native language. We must continue to pray for them. Prayer is the key that will tear down the strongholds of Satan and make people receptive to the wooing of the Holy Spirit. Prayer changes everything because God hears and answers the prayers of His children according to His will. Therefore, "We will give ourselves continually to prayer, and to the Ministry of the Word." (Acts 6:4) We will see others saved!

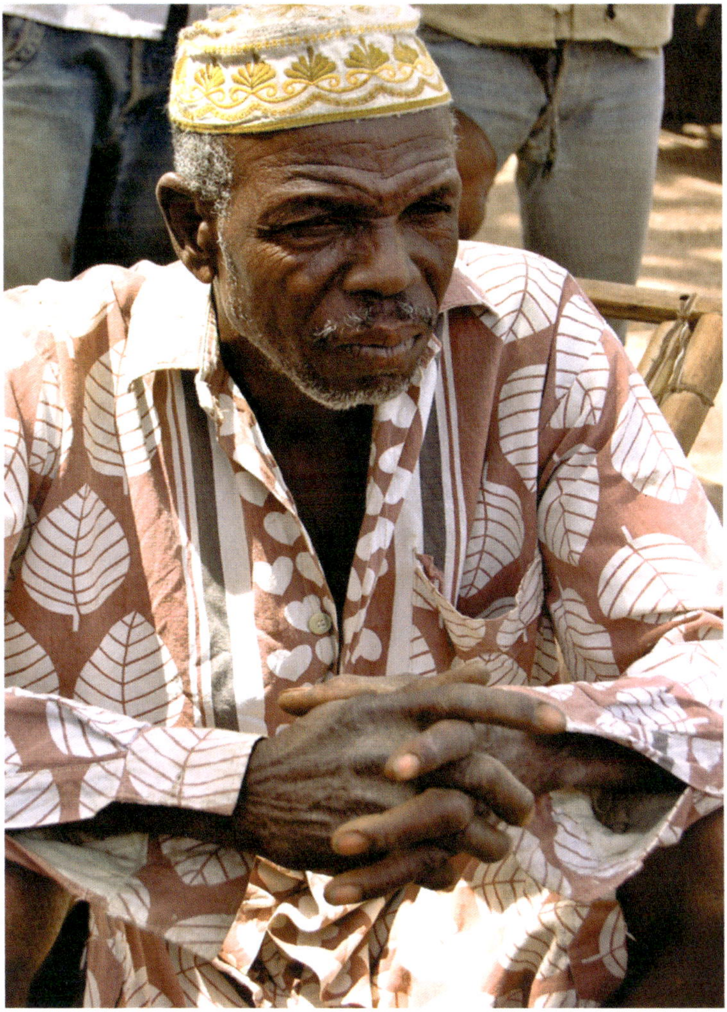

The Village King Angered By The Word

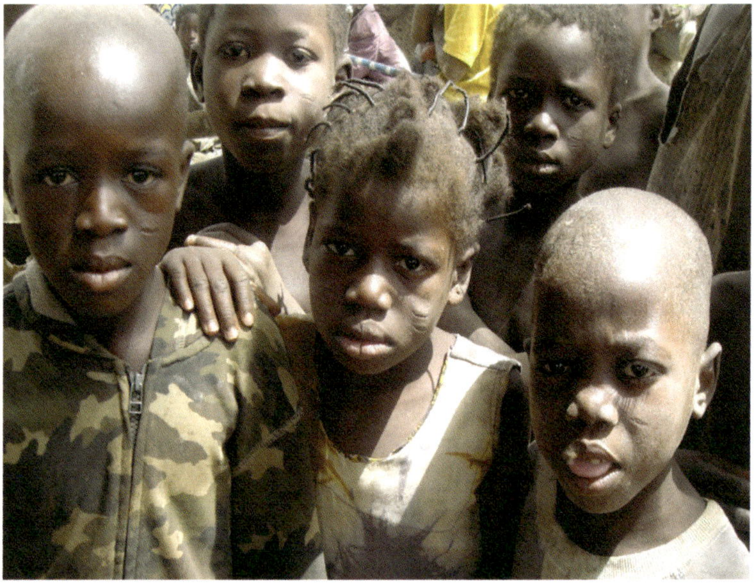

African Faces With An Invitation--- Help!

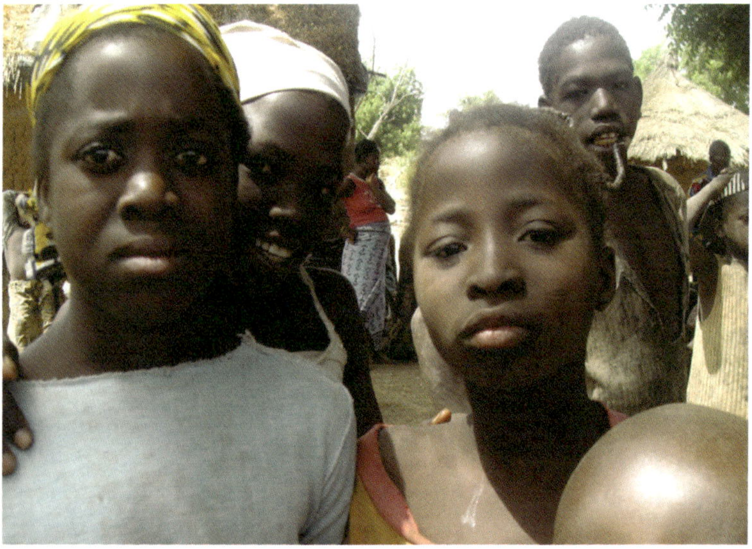

A COINCIDENCE OR A GOD THING?

February 16

Mike originally did not plan for the wound care teams to go out into the villages but for some reason he changed his mind and wanted a team to return to this particular village. My understanding was that one of the wound care teams had visited the village earlier in the week but Mike was led to send a team back one more time. Mike told Dane to gather up a team and go. I volunteered of course and so did 12 other people.

Nionon was the name of the village. Pastor Ag would be our preacher and Samuel would do the interpreting. The van was packed as might be expected with 13 people whom I mostly did not know. We drove a short distance of about 2 or 3 miles over the worst road imaginable. We were so tightly packed inside that one barely noticed the bumpy ride. I suppose we cushioned each other.

We arrived at the village. Pastor Ag and Samuel went to find the chief while the rest of us just looked around. There was a school across the road from the village. Five villages in the area sent their children to this school. A beautiful woman saw our van and came over to greet us. She introduced herself as Elise. She was a missionary to Nionon and had been teaching at the school for 5 years. She also covered the village of Enocule. She was to be in Nionon on this particular day. As she was speaking, Casey realized he had met her before. He asked her a couple of questions and when Casey was assured he had indeed once met her, it became an emotional reunion.

Casey told me the story behind his first encounter with Elise. Casey had been part of the construction team two years ago. He had some down time so he decided to play with the children in the area. He had recruited a young boy by the name of Yaw-yaw to help him teach the kids some games. It was around 10:00 in the morning when a young teenage boy approached Casey and asked him to go to the church. Casey did not feel he could do that at the time and told him so. The teenage boy was persistent and returned several times over the course of 4 hours. Around 2:00 p.m. when the teenager returned, Casey decided he would go see what was so urgent at the church. Almost as an afterthought, Casey asked Yaw-yaw to go with him.

They found the church. Casey went inside and sat in the back. Elise was sitting in the front of the church praying and singing praises to God. At some point she realized Casey was there and went back to meet him. She told him that God had told her to go to the church. She did not know why she needed to be there other than she was convinced God wanted her to go to the church. She had been at the church since early morning praying and singing and waiting on God to show her why she was to be there and on that particular day.

I am uncertain of all the details that transpired from that point but Yaw-yaw accepted Christ as Savior. Elise was called by God to go to the church and pray and the young teenage boy was the messenger to get Casey and Yaw-yaw to the church so that he might be saved. Yaw-yaw just happened to be the chief of the village youngest son. The chief was Muslim.

Casey said that this reunion with Elise must have been the reason why he was to go with the wound team that day. It was a sweet reunion with memories of a young boy giving his heart to the Lord and the woman who prayed.

Pastor Ag came back to the group after meeting the chief of Nionon. The chief wanted us to come back later that night because most of the villagers were gone to market or the fields. Pastor Ag told him that we would not be able to come back later because we would be packing to leave. The chief was not happy with the information. He said for us to go the next village down the road. The village was about ¼ mile away. The team packed-up our supplies and walked to the next village.

I was walking on the dirt path toward the village with Samuel close by. He got my attention and pointed to a small grove of trees that sat off the road about 100 yards. The grove of trees sat on top of a knoll and the trees were very dense. Someone passing by would not be able to see through the forest. Samuel told me that this was a sacred forest called Koulbilou where villagers practiced their fetish religion and worshipped the fetish gods. He also said that gold had been discovered in the forest but it was not mined. The grove of trees looked like any ordinary grove of trees but what was practiced inside that forest was not ordinary or good.

We arrived at the village. Very few people were there. The village looked the same as other African villages but it had a run-down appearance and it looked dirty. It is difficult to make dirt look dirtier or for dirt to look clean but some villagers did make their huts and surroundings look clean. A man named Pale´ (pronounced Pauley) Konote came with us on our trip. Pale´ was from this village called Jnonan. He was a friendly man who had a big smile on his face all the time. He was a pastor/evangelist in Doropo and he showed us around the village.

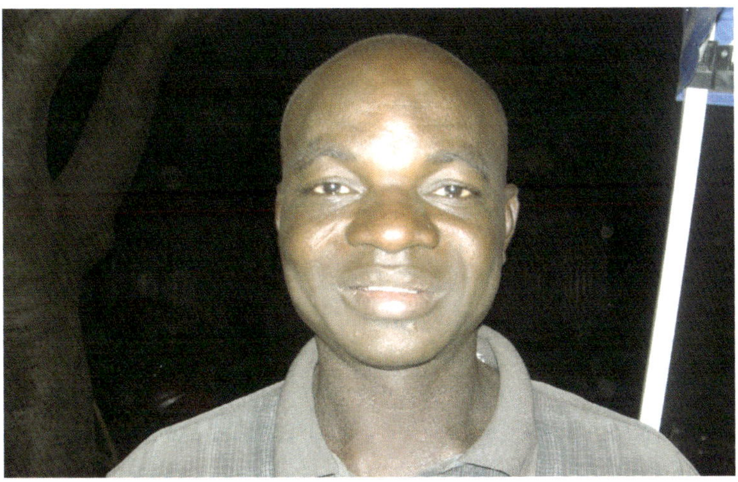

Pastor Pale´

Pale´ took us to the town center where a large concrete slab laid. He said that was the grave of his father and his mother was buried on the outskirts of the village. His father had been the chief. He said that he was to succeed his father's position when he died but Pale´ was a Christian and this disqualified him from becoming chief of the village. Pale´ showed us the baobab tree where he was married and the house where he and his wife first lived. He was a very pleasant man.

I do not know who received permission for Pastor Ag to preach the Good News and for us to give wound care, but we proceeded as planned. We gathered under a shade tree and Pastor Ag preached the Good News as Samuel interpreted. There were only seven adults present for the preaching but there were twice as many children. Unfortunately, to my knowledge, no one accepted Christ as Savior.

Wound care started after the preaching stopped. Several children needed their scrapes attended to. Nothing out of the ordinary was seen until a young woman named Bini appeared on the scene. Her right hand had been bandaged and she acted as if she were in pain. Someone from the wound care team unwrapped her hand and what a medical site to behold. The back of her hand had an approximate 3-4 centimeter open wound that was oozing pus. Her hand was swollen but it was apparent her hand had been swollen twice its size by the loose skin surrounding the wound. Her middle finger and ring finger had an open abscess that channeled to the wound on the back of her hand. She turned her hand over to expose the palm. There was a 2-3 centimeter open wound that was pus filled. The infection from the wound on the back of her hand eroded through to the palm. She needed immediate attention but not from the wound care team. She was too sick.

I had no intention of offering my medical opinion throughout the week as I traveled with the wound care team unless asked. However, being a nurse for 40 years and a nurse who was well experienced in wound care, I spoke up and said she needed to go to the hospital. I believed all of us knew that but we also knew the hospital and the doctors were shutting down at noon and it was 11:00 a.m. There would be no guarantee the doctors would be able to see her due to the time frame. I believed it was Dane who called Mike and told him what the situation was. The next thing I knew, a note was written for her to see the nurse at the hospital to be evaluated. They told her to get to the hospital ASAP and even if she went, she may not be seen. We stressed the importance of getting treatment else she could lose her hand, arm, or possibly her life. She stood and went her way. We were hopeful she would go to the hospital and we were prayerful that the doctors would be able to treat her wounds.

It was time to leave the village. The wound care team packed-up their supplies and we ventured back to the van. As we were leaving the village, two women approached Jordan and me and wanted us to take their babies. The babies looked sick with sunken eyes, runny noses, and the absence of superficial body fat. They looked extremely malnourished, weak, and with failure to thrive syndrome. Perhaps they were infected with HIV. Obviously, Jordan and I could not take the babies with us. I also doubted if the babies would live to see next year.

I was sad to leave the village. I loved going with the wound care team who were so capable and caring. But all good things must come to an end—until next year, God willing.

We arrived back at camp. I immediately went to the OR (operating room) to find my husband. I wanted to tell him that we had sent a woman from the village to the hospital that needed surgery and IV antibiotics. I found him in the OR where he and Dr. Jay were ending a case. I told Dale that he *had* to see this patient and do surgery if at all possible. He said they would do the patient if they could but one OR had already been shutdown and Dr. Jay would have to make that call as well. Not one to easily take no for an answer, I said something to the effect, "You have to. God sent us to that village just for her."

Guilt trips can be effective but this situation did not need any help. I told Dale that the wound care team had visited the village earlier in the week but the woman was not seen and for some reason, Mike sent us back. It was a God thing that needed to be taken care of!

I then left the OR and went to triage to check if Bini had made it to the hospital. There she sat! She had made it to the hospital and was being evaluated by the nurse. I ran back to the OR and told my husband that the patient was on the premises and to not shut-down the OR. He gave me one of those familiar looks I had seen many times in our 37 years of marriage. I was not scared. Then out of the blue he said he needed to run and get something to eat and drink while the patient was being evaluated. As he "wolfed down" his peanut butter and crackers at the camp dining room, Sabrina showed up and asked if he would be willing to do the hand on the girl we sent in. (For clarity, Dale is not a surgeon but an anesthesiologist. He would be giving the anesthesia so the surgeon could perform the surgery.) Of course he would be willing—he just wanted to make sure other medical personnel would be available.

Less than an hour later, Bini was in surgery. I went back to the OR to watch and assist if needed. I helped place Bini on the table and I thought she would recognize me since I had seen her just two hours earlier. She acted like she did not recognize me and perhaps it was because of the hat I was wearing. It made me think how awful it would be to go to surgery and not know the doctors or nurses or anything about the procedure, what to expect, or even the complications of anesthesia. Communication could not be optimal because of the language barrier and word meaning often gets lost in translation. It would be a very frightful situation.

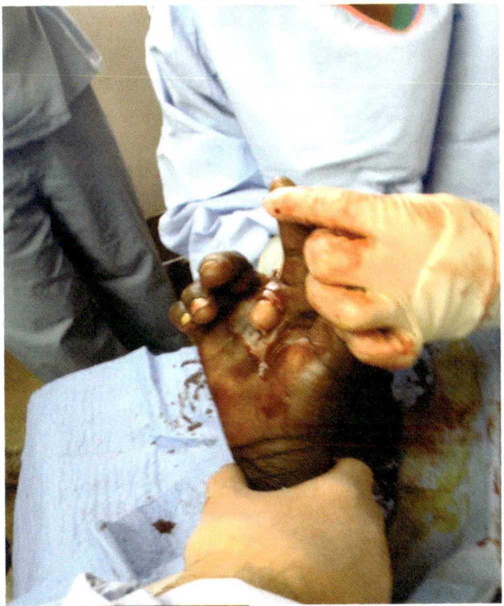

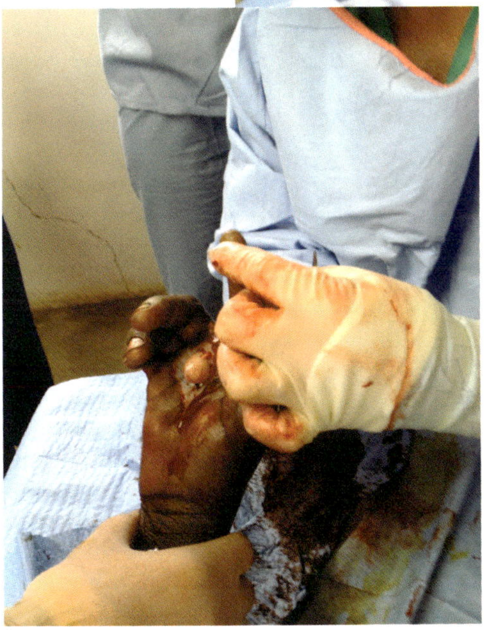

Dr. Jay Performing Surgery On Bini's Hand. Notice Dr. Jay's Finger Protruding From The Back Of The Hand Into The Palm.

Dr. Jay began the surgical procedure of an I & D (incision and drainage) on the wound. During the procedure, Dr. Jay was able to stick his thumb through the wound on the back of her hand through to the palm. He packed it with sterile gauze and said that she should be all right if she took care of the wound. That seemed like a big IF considering her living conditions and environment. Dale gave Bini two strong IV antibiotics for the infection and she was taken to Post-op for monitoring. Later, I stuck my head in the Post-op tent and she was awake, alert, and nursing her baby. All in a day's work!

I was thankful for Mike and his sensitivity to the Holy Spirit's leading him to send the wound care team to the previously visited village. Bini had been overlooked for some reason and God wanted her to be seen. One can only speculate how God will use this situation to bring glory to Him. A follow-up visit will be in order for next year—perhaps she will be a believer by then!

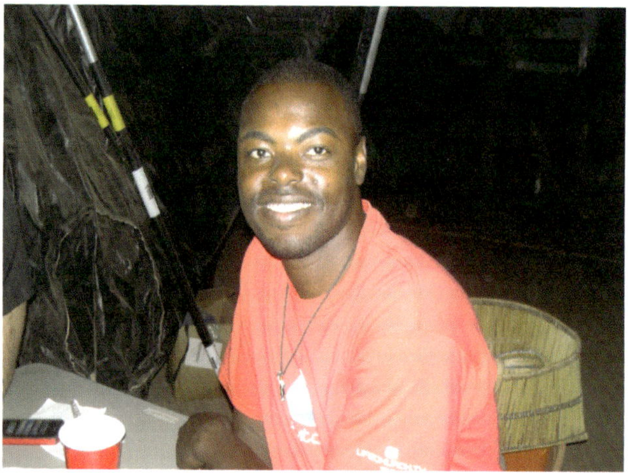

Samuel
My Interpreter And Friend

PALE´ AND THE DEMONIAC BROTHER

Pale´ (pronounced Pauley) was an interesting African man with a very interesting past. I regretted I did not get to meet him until late in our stay at Camp Doropo because he had quite the story. He was well acquainted with the evil manifestations of the fetish religion but he was also fully aware of the almighty power of God over evil. He witnessed God tear down the strongholds of Satan over his family that brought them into a relationship with Christ.

Pale´ attended a Free Will Baptist Church as a child. His parents did not object that he attended a Christian church at that time but they wanted no part of the Christian faith. They would remain devout worshippers of the fetish gods of their culture. A man by the name of Joseph was his pastor and Joseph had worked closely with the missionaries in that area. Pale´ enjoyed attending the Christian church. He learned about God, the Bible, and heard Bible stories. The seed of faith had been planted in his heart at a young age.

When Pale´ became a teenager, his parents prevented him from attending the Christian church and required him to practice the cultural religion. He was getting old enough to take on the responsibilities of fetish worship. However, he despised the fetish religion. He felt like a slave—enslaved to idolatry. He said there were many superstitions about the religion and one had to believe many things just to worship the fetish gods. All the time he was forced to practice the fetish religion, his thoughts would take him back to the Free Will Baptist Church he attended as a child. He desired to return there one day.

Pale´ lived in his father's village 25 years and would be considered the next chief of the village. He was married and also old enough to decide what religion he wanted to practice. He chose Christianity and this choice prevented him succeeding his father as chief of the village. He started attending an Assembly of God Church nearby because at the time, there were no Free Will Baptist Churches near his village. Pale´ was saved, September 27, 1989 in the Assembly of God Church in Gagnoa and later baptized in 1990. Pale´ said that he wanted freedom from the fetish gods he had known as a child and had found it with Christ.

I asked Pale´ how difficult was it to follow Christ? How did Christianity impact his life? Pale´ said that once he became a Christian, his family would no longer come around. He became an outcast to his family and community. He also mentioned that once his wife's family became aware of his Christianity, they came to his house and took his wife back home. His marriage became invalid.

I asked Pale´ how did he become a Christian? Who showed him? He said that he remembered some of the things from going to church as a child. He said the pastor told him that he would become a new creature in Christ if he gave his heart to Him. Pastor John Liga showed him how to be a Christian and he had also baptized him. Pastor Liga is now the pastor of the Assembly of God Church in Abidjan.

I also asked Pale´ what convinced him that God was different from the fetish gods? Pale´ said everything was different from God and the fetish gods. With God there was freedom. He said that the Truth had sat him free and God was the Truth. He had freedom from the fetishes and freedom from sin. He also stated that he despised taking part in the fetish sacrifices and that it was difficult to believe all the things that go with the religion. It really did not make any sense to him.

Pale´ had such a beautiful smile as he told me those things. He seemed so incredibly happy! I then asked him how his life changed with Christ. He said, "I have joy, peace, and freedom!" I have been set free from the bondage of cultural idolatry. My joy is unspeakable! And I have a new family!

Pale´ is now an evangelist and visits five villages each week. He said that he saw approximately 50 people in each village. Most of the villages he visits are now believers especially in the village of Varale. They believed in God—not that there was a god but a real God that they could confess their sins to. All of the villagers had invited Christ into their hearts. The villagers were now new creatures in Christ.

Pale´ said that even when attending the Assembly of God Church he wanted to be in the Free Will Baptist Church because it was home—where it all really began.

I asked if any of his family were now believers. He said that after his first wife returned back to her home he later remarried a woman who was a believer. He then told me this fascinating story how salvation came to other family members.

As the story goes: Pale´'s uncle was the fetish priest in his village where the python snake was worshipped. There was a special time of the year when the python "visited" the village and the villagers worshipped the serpent. After Pale´ accepted Christ, the python did not come into the village. That started the spiritual warfare between fetish gods and Christianity. The python would not return to the village as long as a Christian was present. Pale´ was accused of running out the idol from the village—the idol the villagers worshipped. As a consequence, Pale´ was asked to leave the village so that the serpent could return.

Pale´'s father had died and of course Pale´ could not become the chief because of his Christianity. Pale´ decided to leave the village and enrolled in the Bible Institute in Bouna. The town was many miles from his village.

His mother continued to practice her fetish worship of the python. Then one day, Pale´ received word from his mother that his brother had gone insane and was living in the sacred forest, a place where fetish worship and sacrifice was performed. He lived naked and would terrorize the villagers or anyone who walked past the forest. He would physically assault people. He was like a wild man.

Pale´'s mother was able to convince her insane son to seek help at a mental institution in Burkina Faso. He was at the institution for a short while but did not get better. His mother then took her son to the fetish idol for healing. His condition only worsened. As Pale´ told me the story I mentioned that the Bible spoke of the demoniac who lived in the tombs, naked, and would terrorize people as they passed by. Pale´ said that was exactly the case with his brother—he was demon possessed.

Pale´ and his friend from the Bible Institute returned to his village. They went into the bush to find his brother. They found him, covered his nakedness and began to pray for him, earnestly, fervently praying that God would heal his brother. In what sounded like a modern day exorcism, the demon left his brother's body and he was healed. The three men returned to the village and everything seemed to be going well for the brother. Pale´ and his friend decided to return to the Bible Institute where they would continue their studies.

Unfortunately, Pale´'s mother returned to her fetish practices and took her son with her to worship the python idol. The son immediately went insane once again. Pale´ heard about the situation with his brother and made another trip back to his village. He took a pastor friend with him. They reached the village and sought out to find Pale´'s brother. This time they took Pale´'s mother with them. They found him in the sacred forest, naked, and acting wild. The pastor and Pale´ prayed for his brother and his mother. In a similar fashion as before, the demon left his brother's body and his brother was healed. The pastor told Pale´'s mother to never pray to the fetish gods again. The fetish gods had caused her son to go insane by demons. When Pale´'s mother saw that her son was healed she realized Pale´'s God was the one true God and more powerful than the fetish gods of idolatry. He had healed her son and Pale´'s mother became a believer!

When Pale´ finished the story, I was in awe. It was like reading a page right out of the Bible on demon possession. Pale´ spoke with such conviction and confidence. He knew the power of God over evil. He had witnessed it in his own family. He had experienced the spiritual warfare of good versus evil and saw the power of the Almighty smite the indwelling evil of Satan and his brother was healed from demon possession. Praise God!

The next morning, the campers at Camp Doropo were loading the bus and truck with their luggage. I was busy helping Dale get our supplies in order when I looked up from my labor and who would be standing next to me but Pale´. He had been trying to locate me before we started our journey home. Pale´ was smiling ear-to-ear and so very happy. Then he said, "I want you to meet someone—my brother—the one who had the demon." Standing next to Pale´ was his brother—the one who was once demon possessed and who lived naked in the sacred forest. He was smiling and colorfully dressed. Pale´ said, "My brother is now a believer!"

Tears were flowing uncontrollably. Nothing could describe the degree of happiness I felt for Pale´ and his brother. I realized I had been privileged to hear about a modern day miracle of the power of God over Satan and his imps of hell. I needed this and to reiterate the statement I wrote in my journal on January 1, 2012: "I want my faith to come alive like never before. I want my heart to feel what my eyes see. I want God to make it real all over again."

I can honestly say God truly did make it real all over again. My heart was quickened by what I saw, heard, touched, and sensed. God is alive and still working miracles today just as He has from the beginning of time. The depth of His love, I cannot understand but am thankful God loved all of us—you know—the world, that He gave His only Son to die on a cross for all sinners. But whoever believes in Him can receive forgiveness and the free gift of eternal life to be enjoyed one day in heaven forever.

I regretted I did not have time to interview Pale´'s brother or even get his name. What a story he would have been able to tell! Perhaps next year if God allows, I will have the opportunity to write the sequel to Pale´'s story about his demoniac brother.

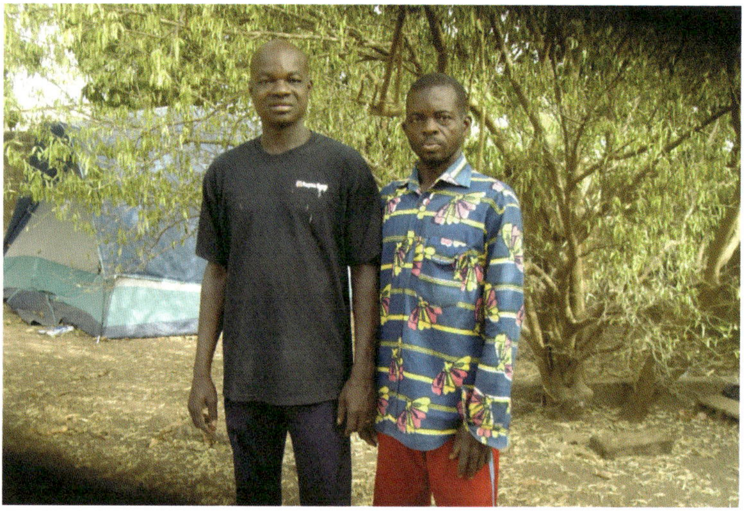

Pale´ And His Brother

I Remember . . .

The Villages

The sight of earth tone villages scattered about the countryside that blended splendidly with the surroundings are deeply etched in my mind. They reflected a simple life but a hard life for those who dwelled within the small communities. The mud brick buildings had a beauty of their own in a rugged sort of way, and the people who made their homes in these earthen structures seemed contented. Young children played happily with no apparent worries about their future. There were no visible signs of manufactured toys to play with—just each other and their imaginations. The villages offered no conveniences. Water was a precious commodity that must be drawn from a well—hopefully, a well within or close to the village. There was no electricity and all chores were done by hand and primitive tools. It was the African way of life that I did not envy, but I felt so privileged to have been part of the experience of helping those with great needs.

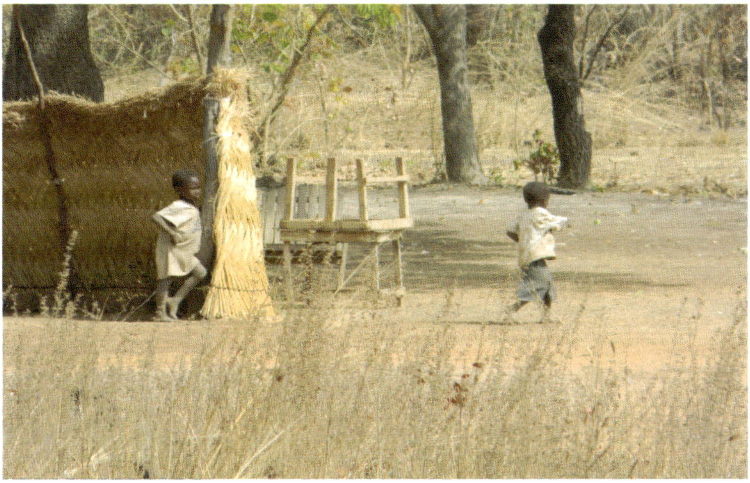

A Common Sight—Children At Play

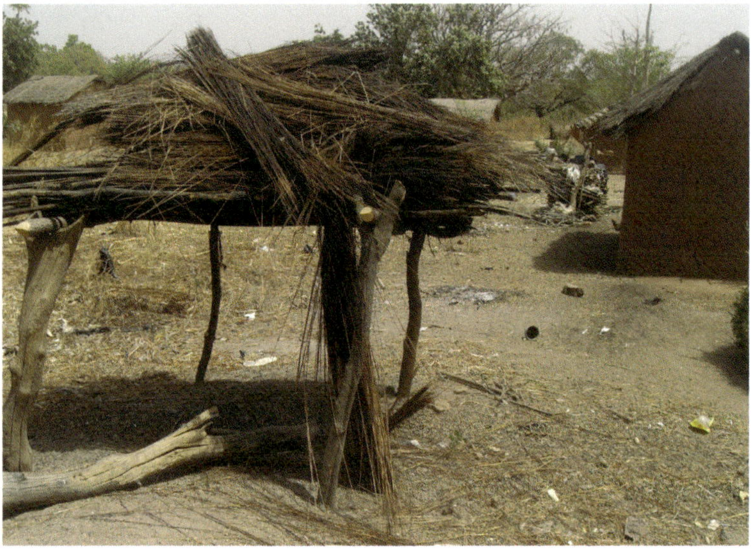

A Place To Escape The African Sun

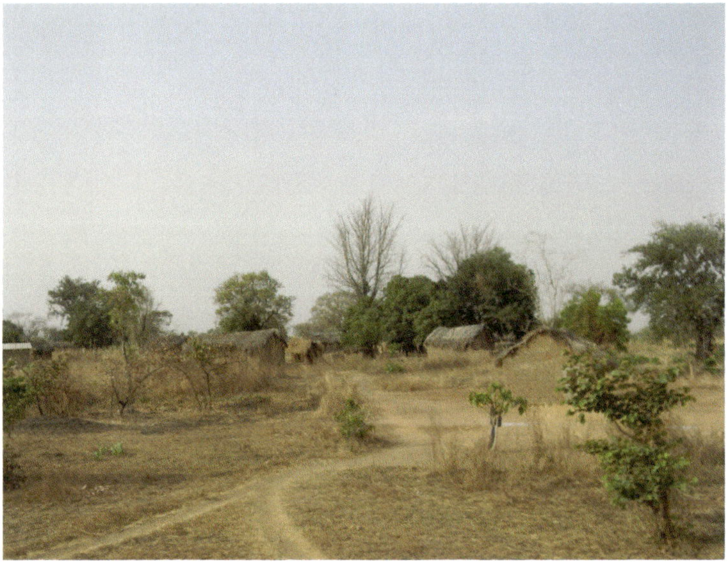

A Peaceful African Village

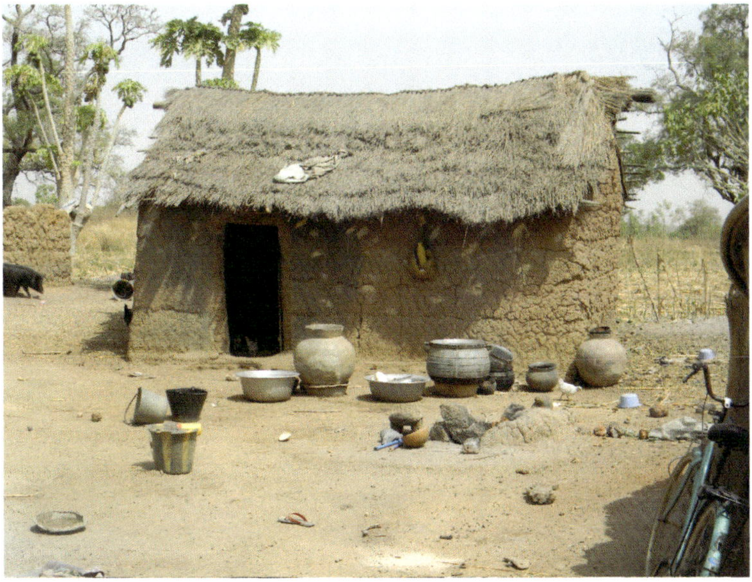

Pots—A Sign Of Wealth

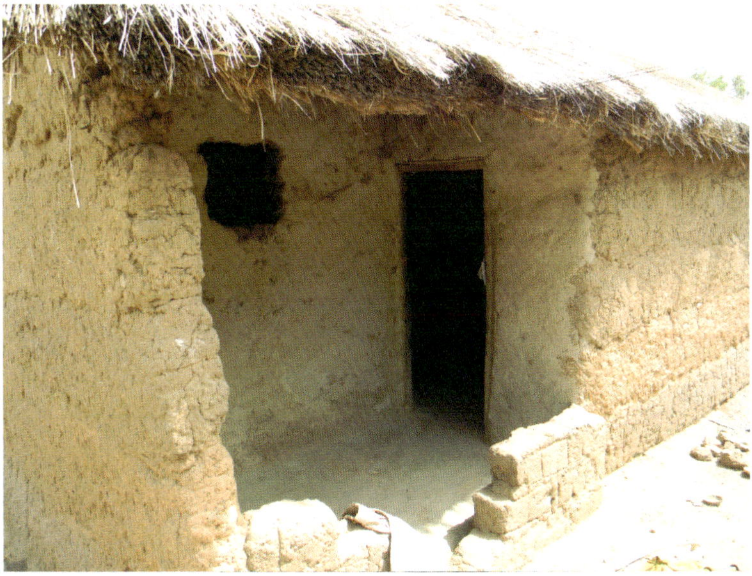

An African Home With A "Porch"

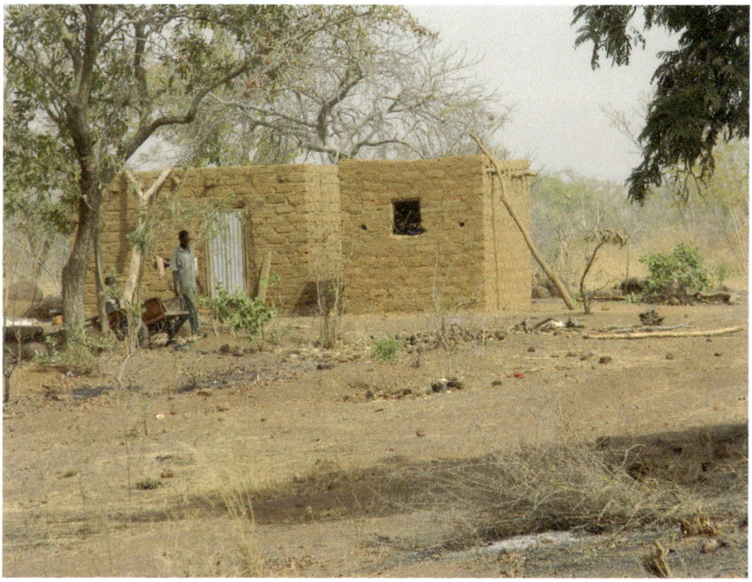

A Typical Mud Brick Home

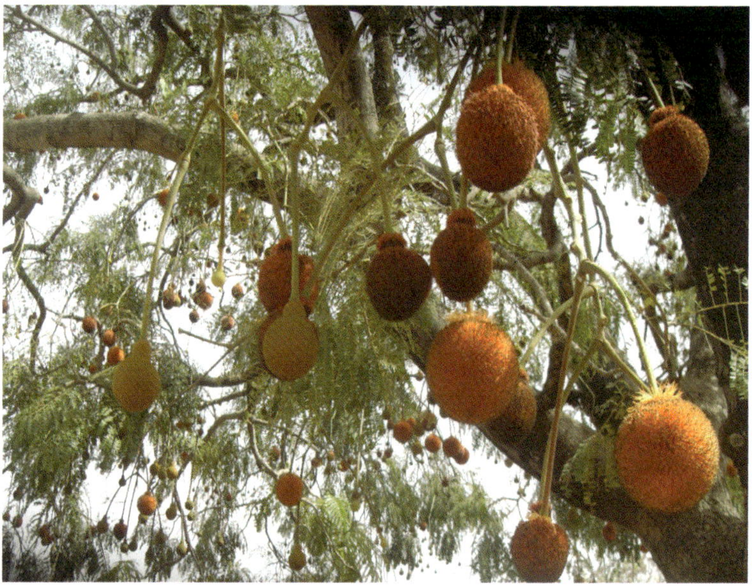

An Unusual Flowering Tree

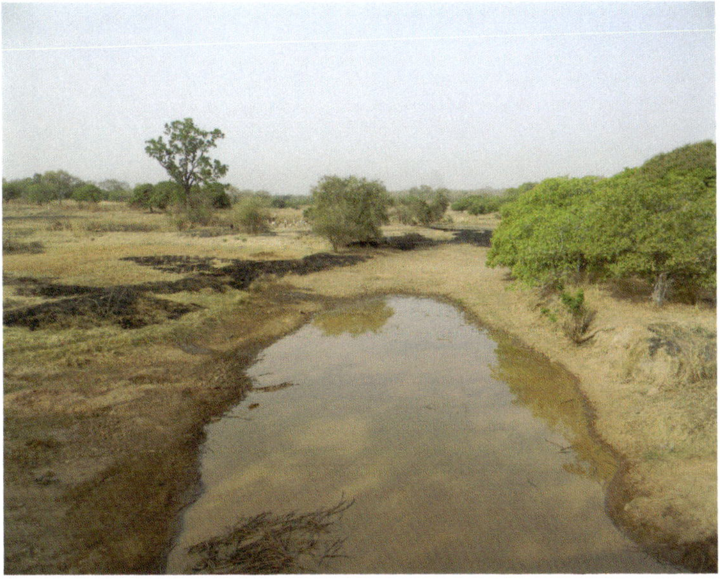

A Contaminated Water Source Where Children Play

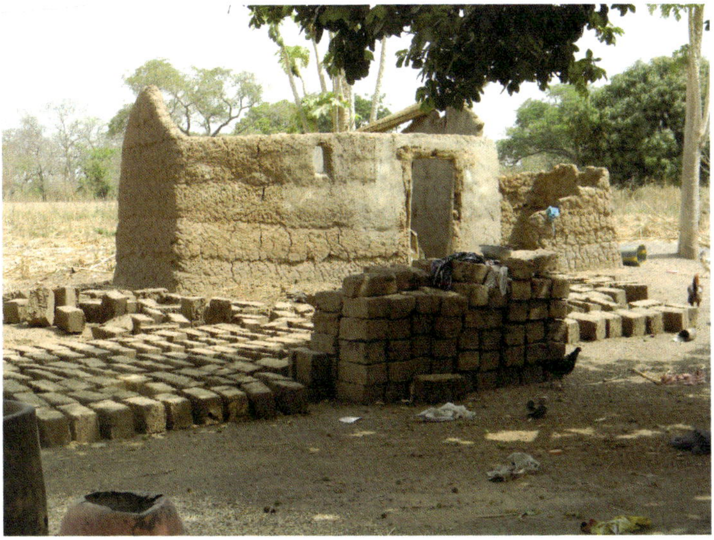

New Brick For A New Building

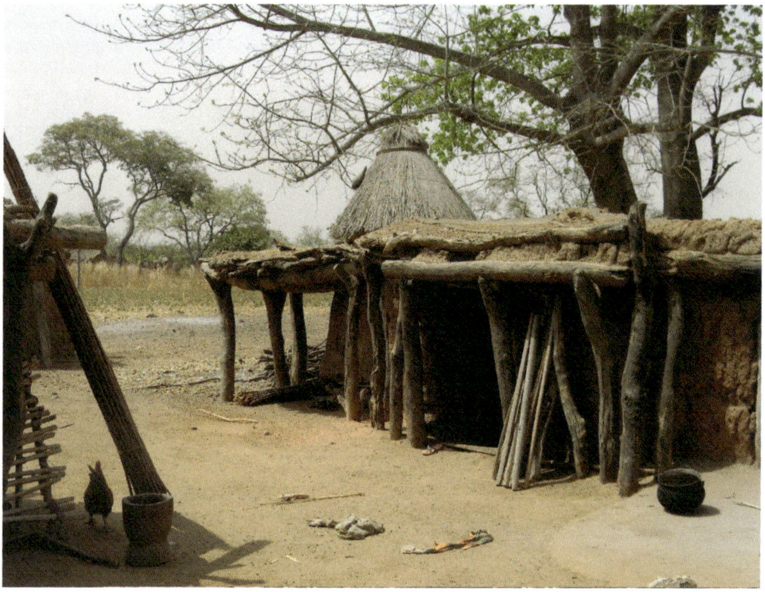

A Family Dwelling

I Remember . . .

The People

It has been said that a picture can paint a thousand words. I believe this is true because volumes could be written about the African people and their way of life from pictures alone: the wrinkled weathered skin of the people from years of exposure; calloused, scarred and disfigured feet from untreated injuries; women gathering water from a community well; so many children with so many needs; health issues created by the environment; aged faces; eyes that had seen and experienced things so painful to remember yet unable to forget; happy faces of children; the smiles of Salvation and knowing God; sadness and uncertainty; and faces of hope. The thousands of words created by pictures filled volumes of unwritten texts in my heart.

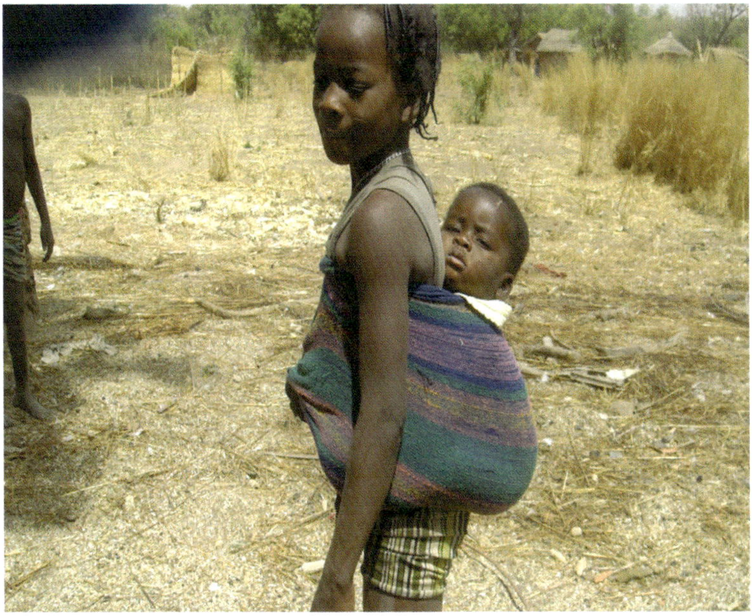

Young Girl Caring For Her Sibling

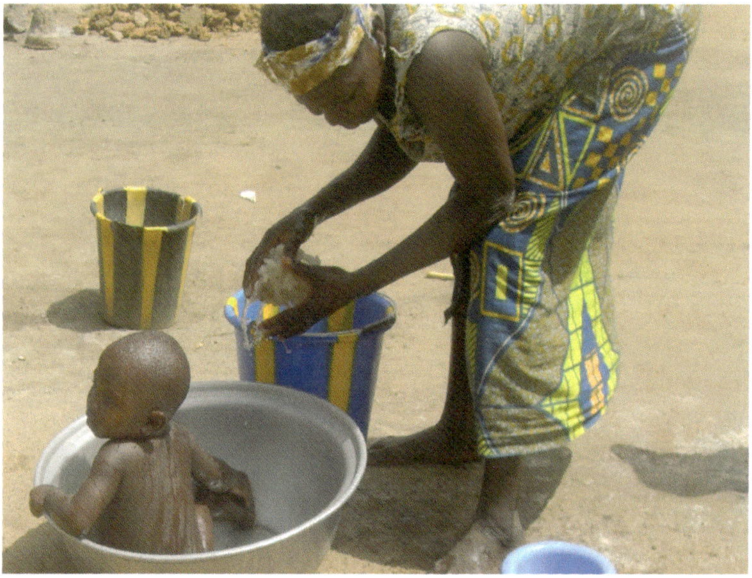

Mother Bathing A Child In One Inch Of Water

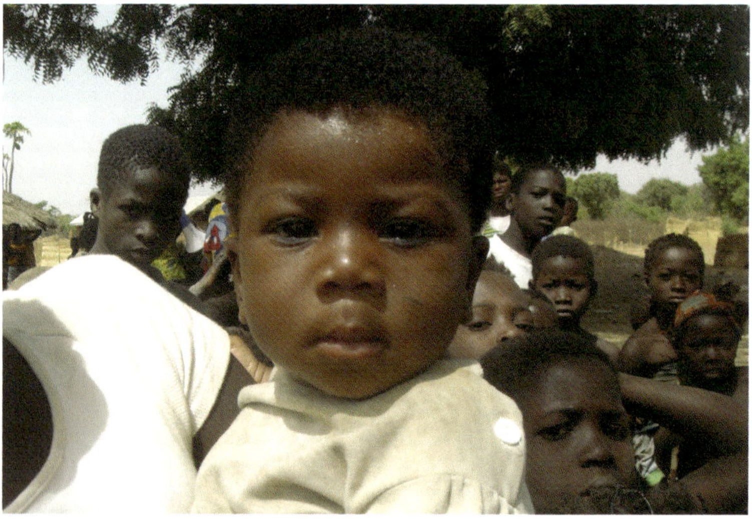

What Does His Future Hold?

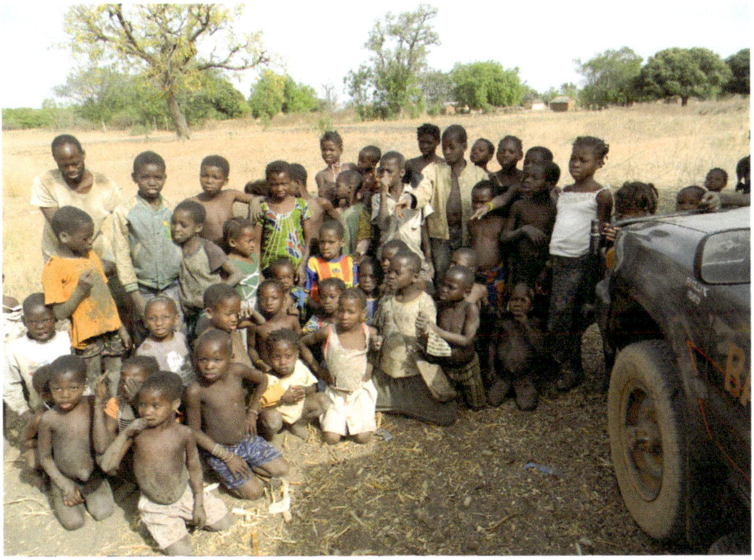

Children Everywhere

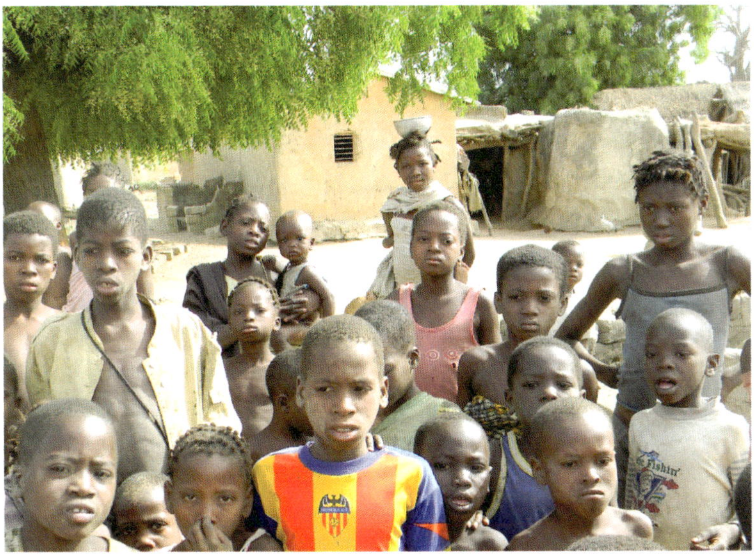

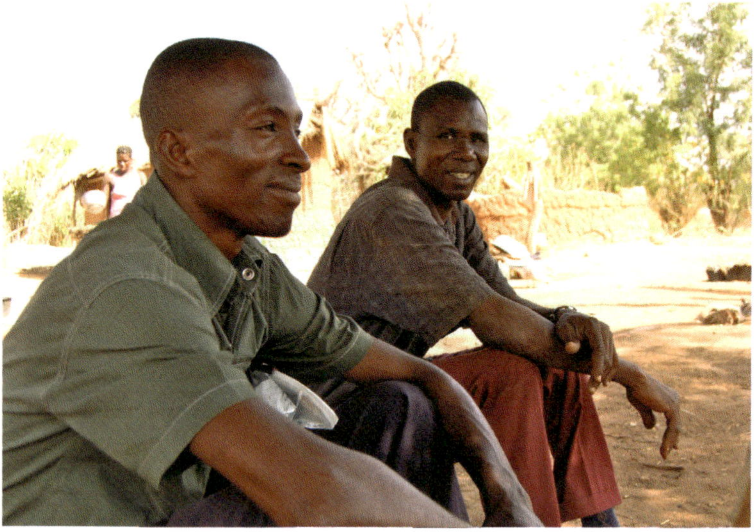

African Men Who Are Believers

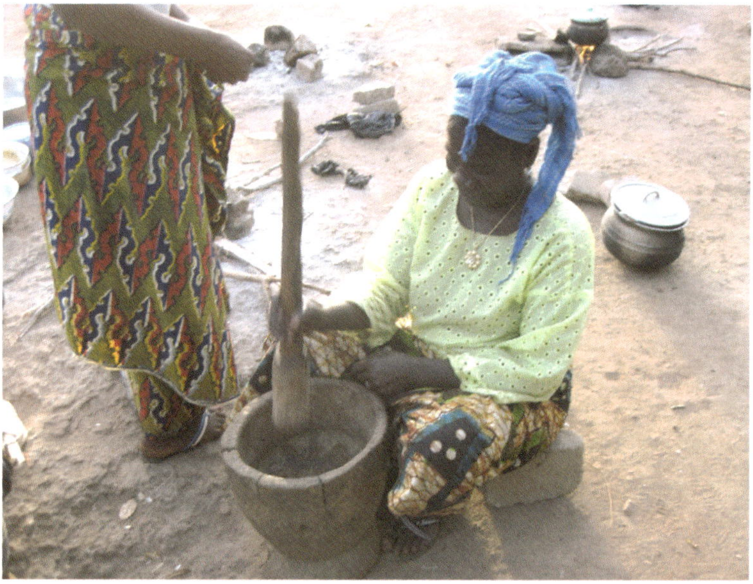

Food Being Prepared For Her Family

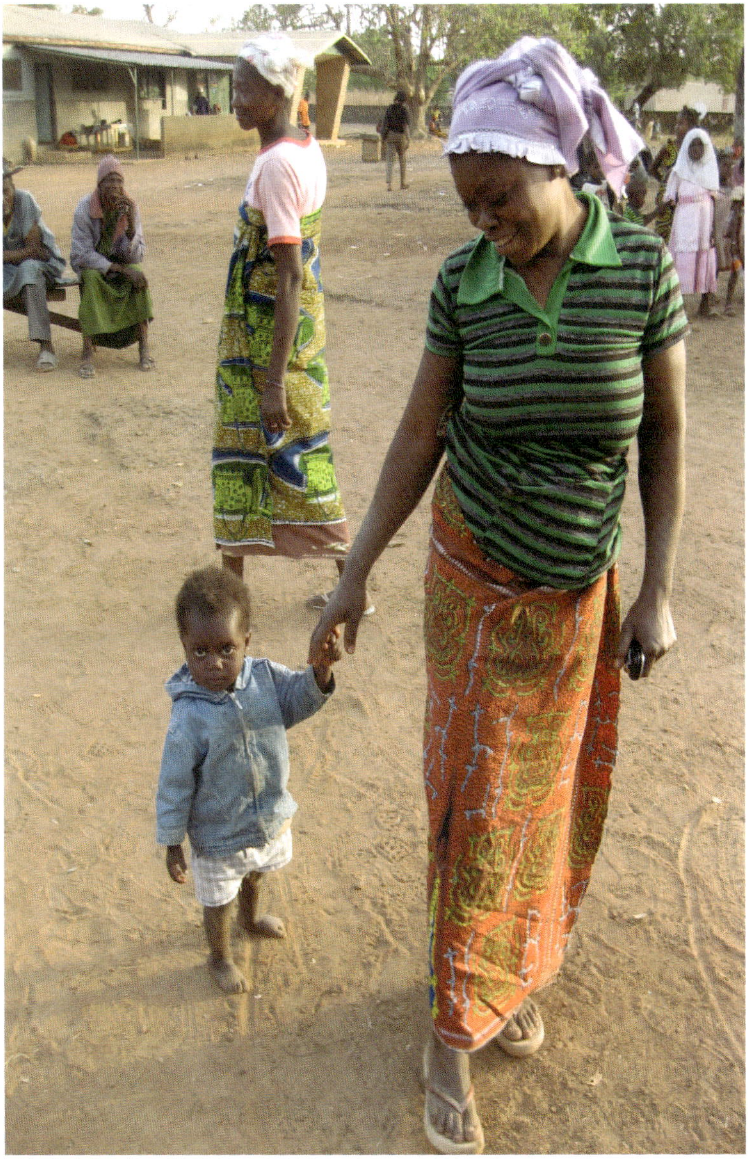

A Skeptical Stare
By A Child Having His Picture Made

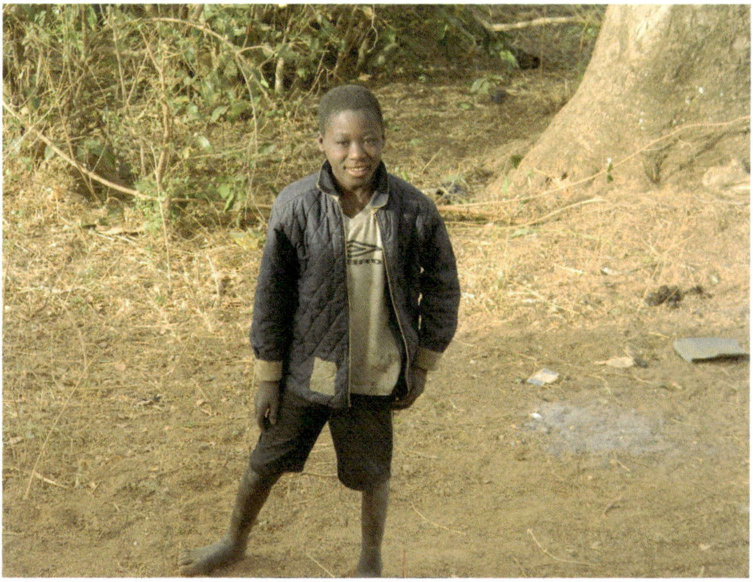

The Sweet Innocence Of Children

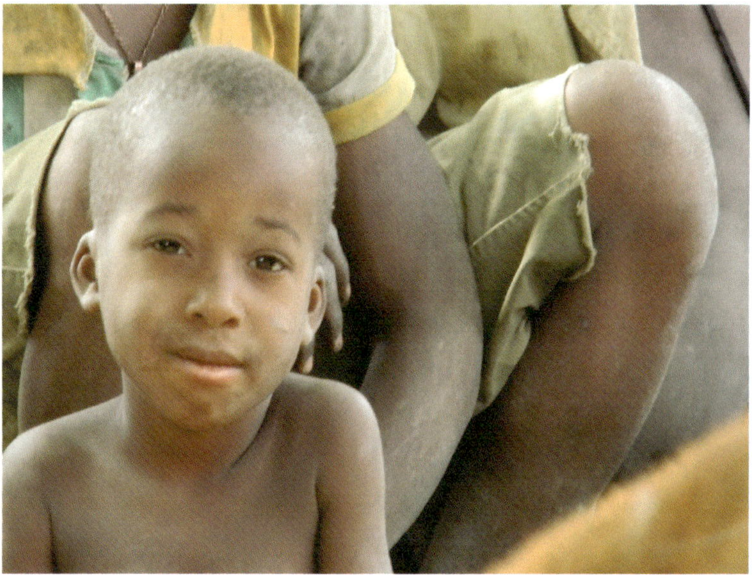

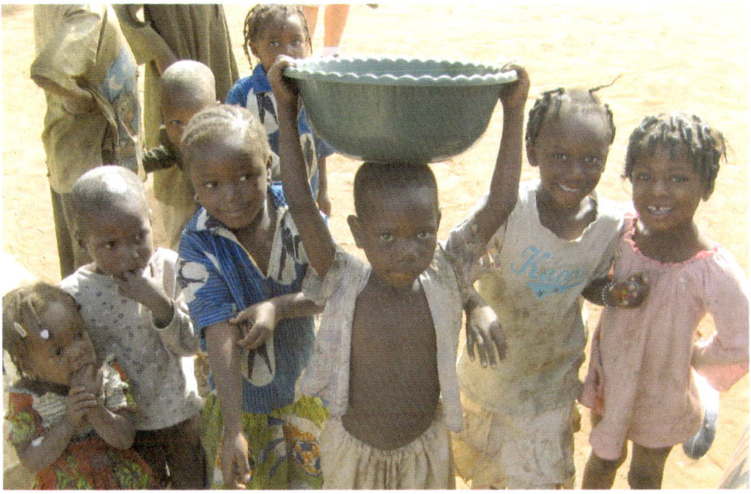

Children Helping With Chores

"Jesus Loves The Little Children
All The Children of the World;
Red and Yellow, Black and White
They Are Precious In His Sight;
Jesus Loves The Little Children
Of The World."

But Jesus said, Suffer little children, and forbid them not, to come unto me: for of such is the kingdom of heaven.
--Matthew 19:14

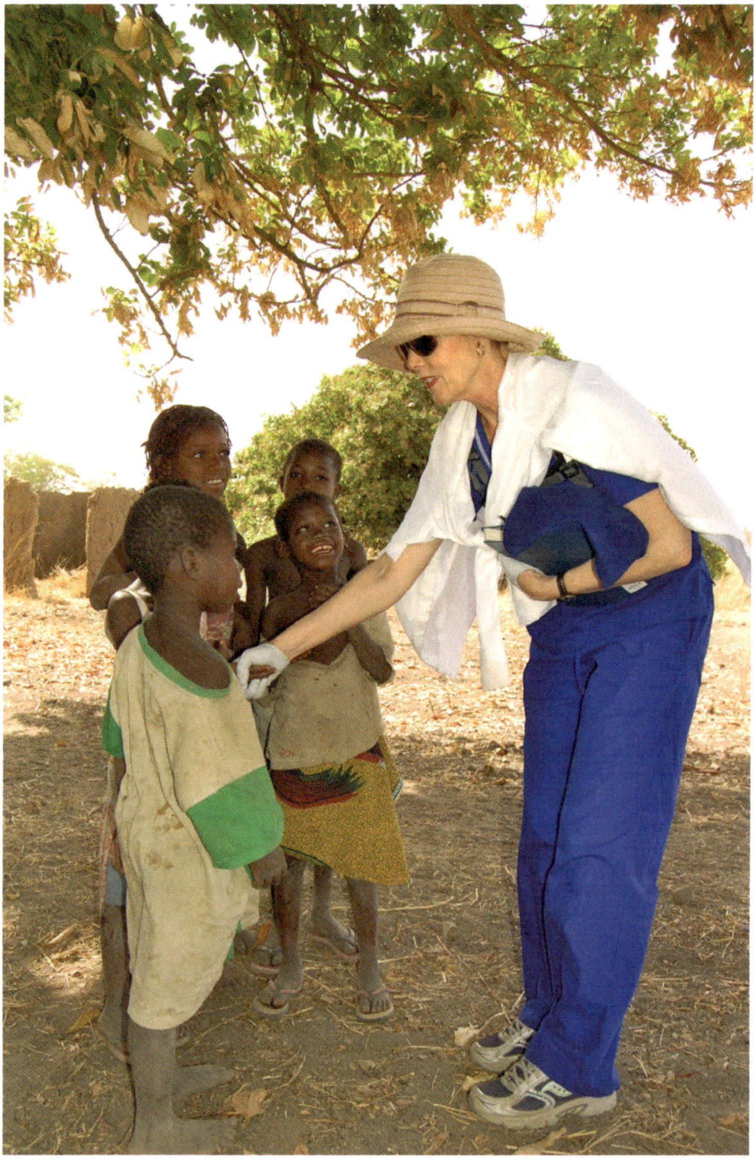

Tangba Nafer—"Jesus Loves You"

I Remember ...

The Medical Needs And The Medical Care

The medical needs of the African people are many. Unfortunately, there was not enough time or resources to treat everyone with medical needs. Those who were treated by the capable medical team received excellent care and for many, the treatment was life changing: A person would no longer be an outcast in their village if a deformity were corrected. Other villagers were given sight and a clear vision of life with glasses. They were not picky about the frames either. Men proudly wore women's glasses if it helped their vision. Children and adults had life-saving surgeries while some received palliative treatment to provide comfort for the inevitable passage of life. The lives that were touched by the healing hands of the medical team also touched the lives of those administering care. We will never forget their faces or their stories.

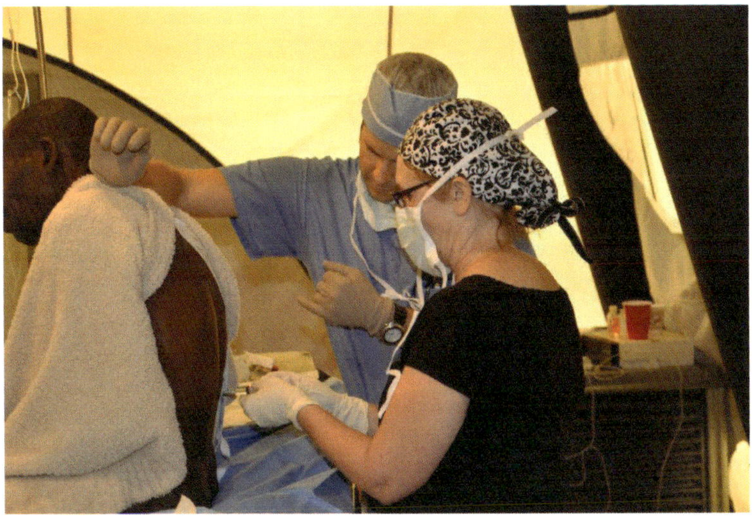

"And heal the sick that are therein, and say unto them, The kingdom of God is come nigh unto you". -Luke 10:9

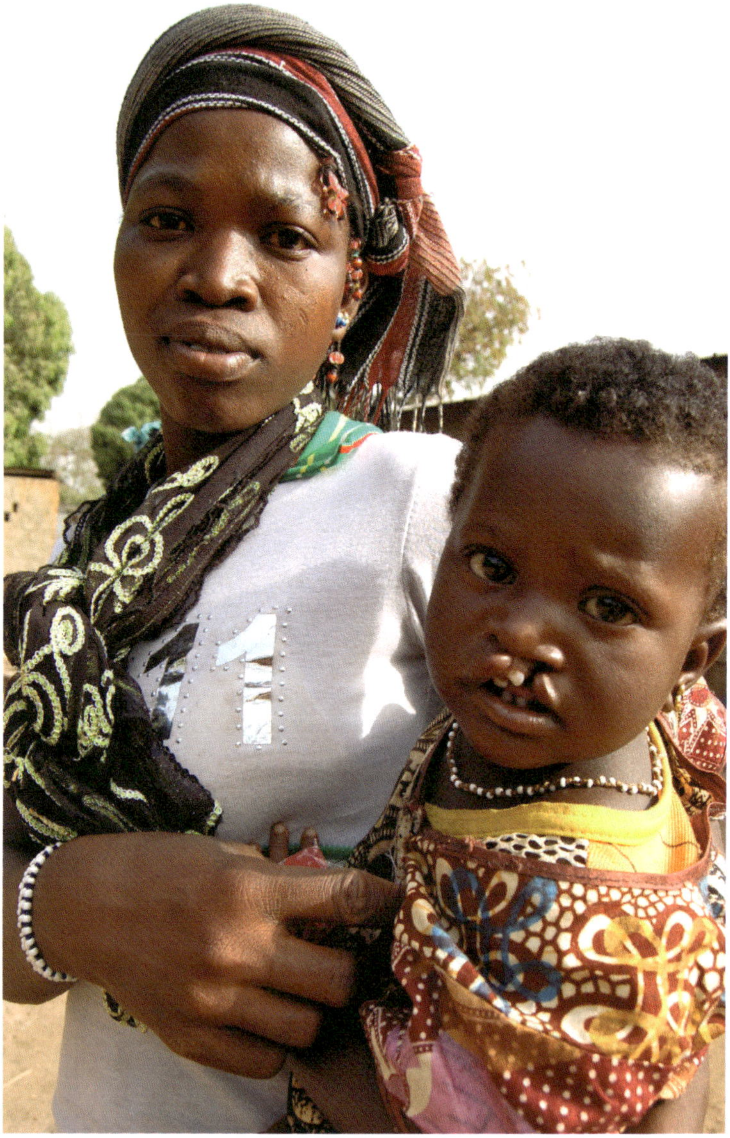

Cleft Lip—A Common Defect Seen
In
African People

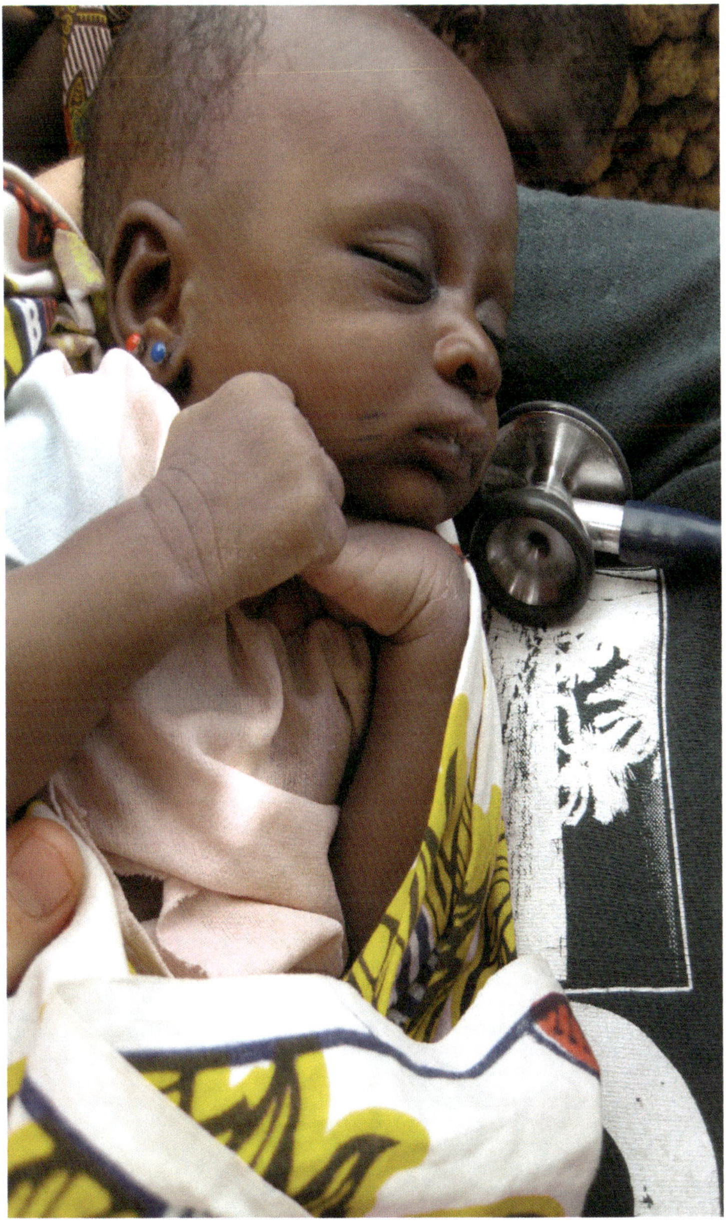

Tiny Child With Two Tribal Markings On Lower Right Cheek

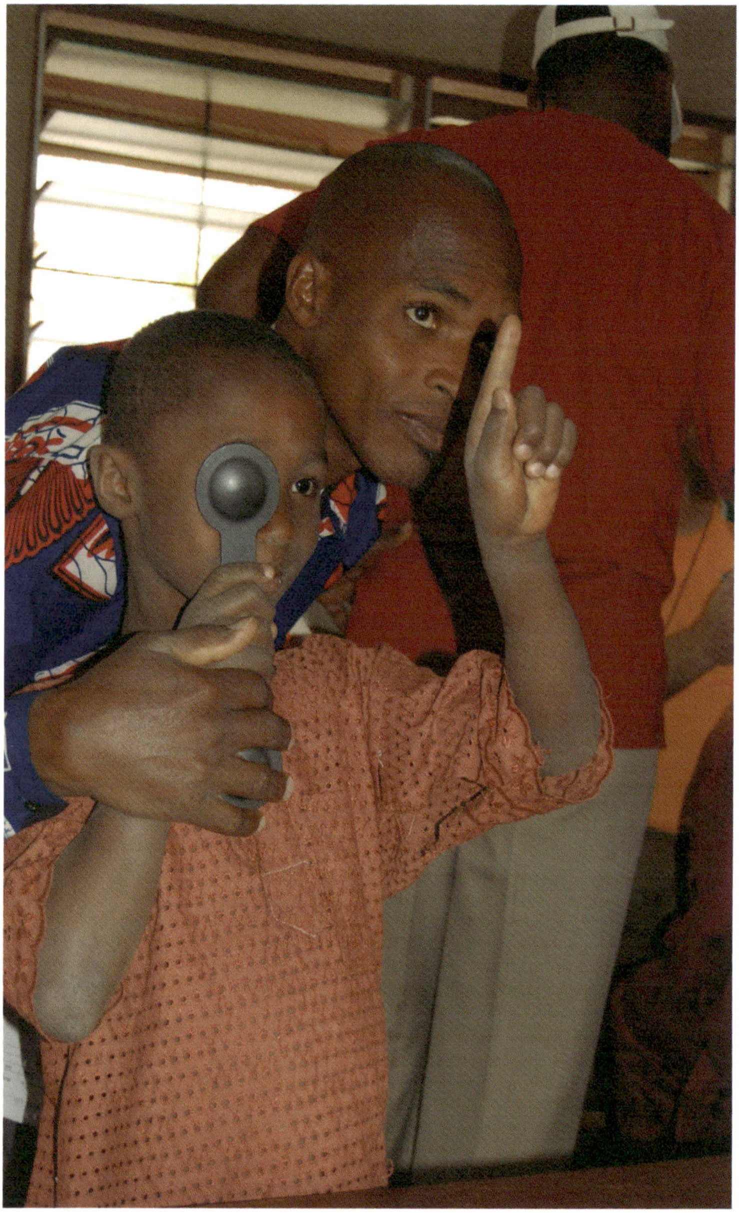

Child Receiving Eye Examination

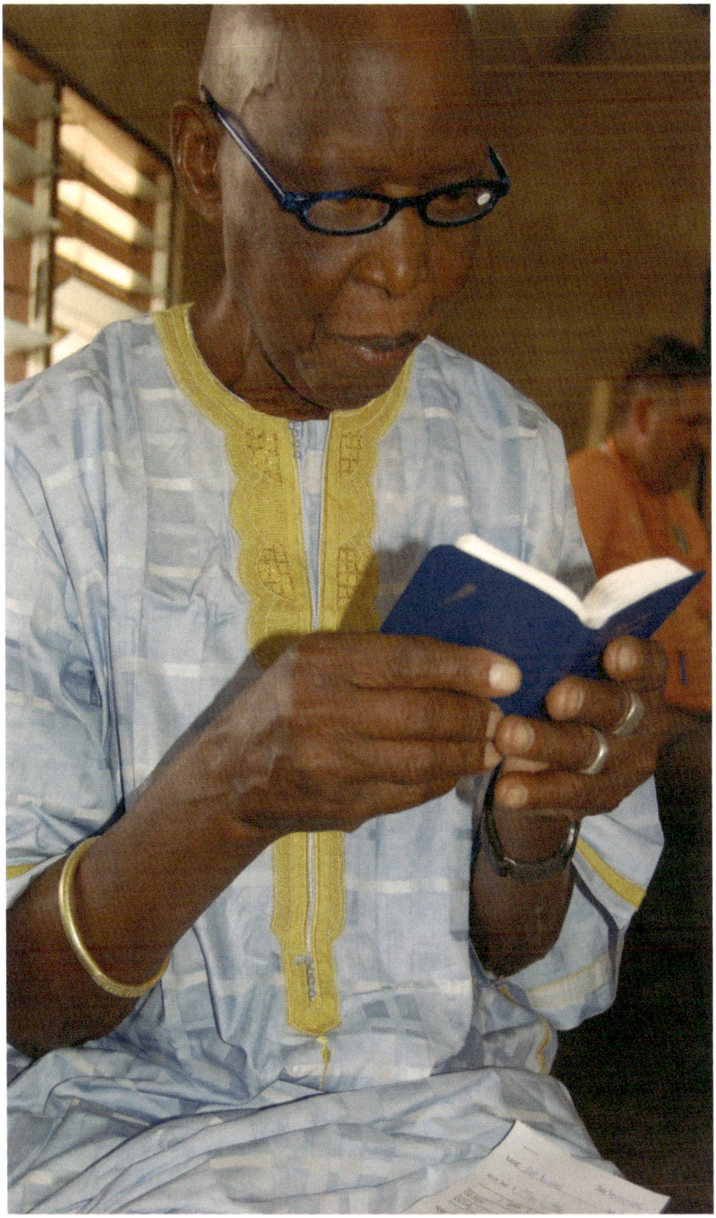

New Glasses To Aid Reading God's Word

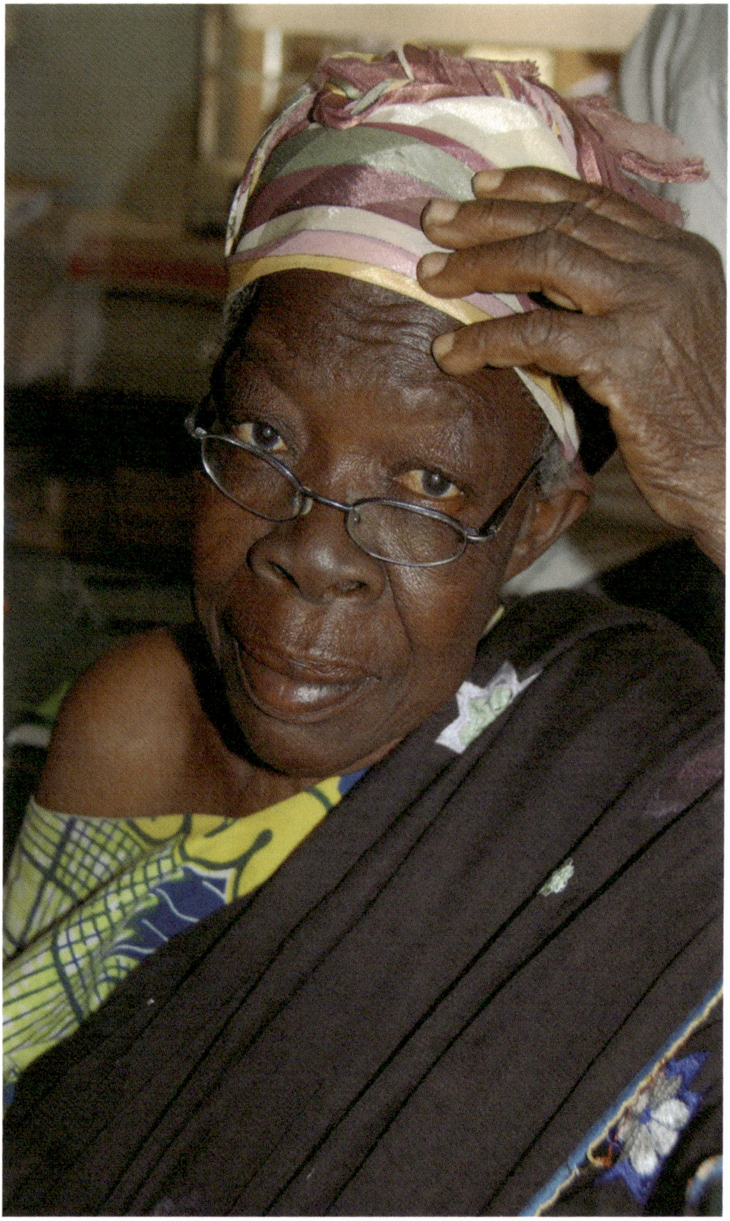

The Smile Of An African Woman With New Glasses

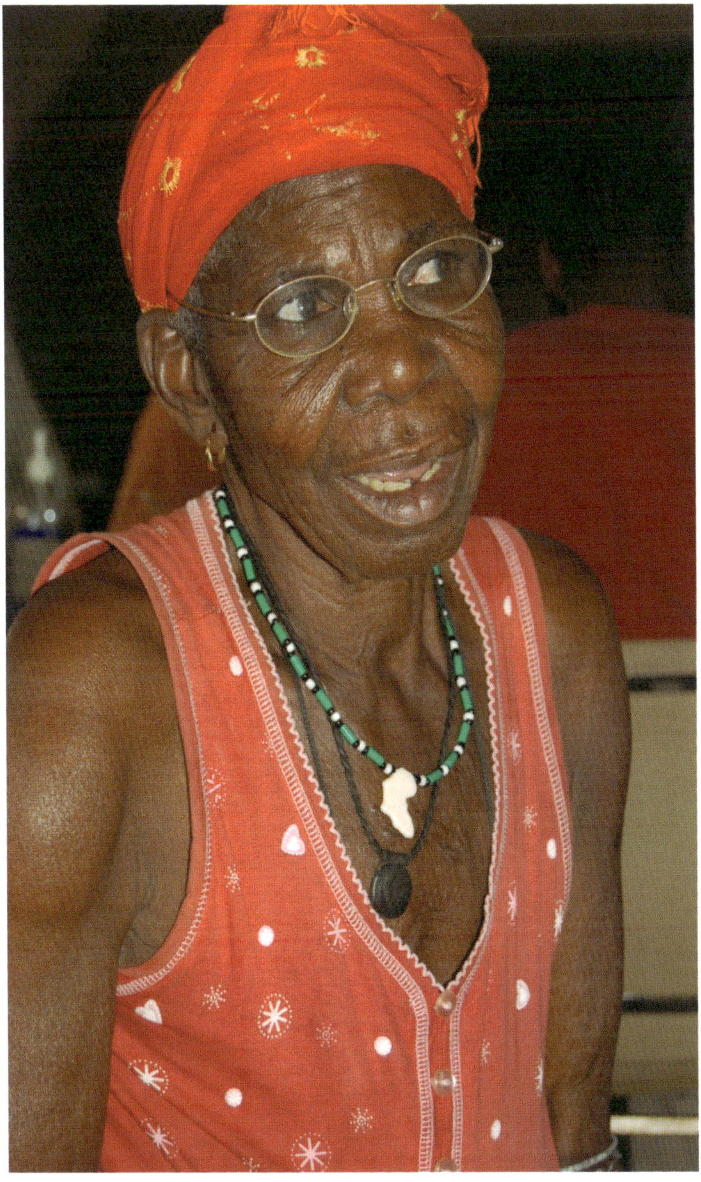

Glasses Will Open-Up A Whole New World For Those With Poor Sight

Micah With A Local Child.

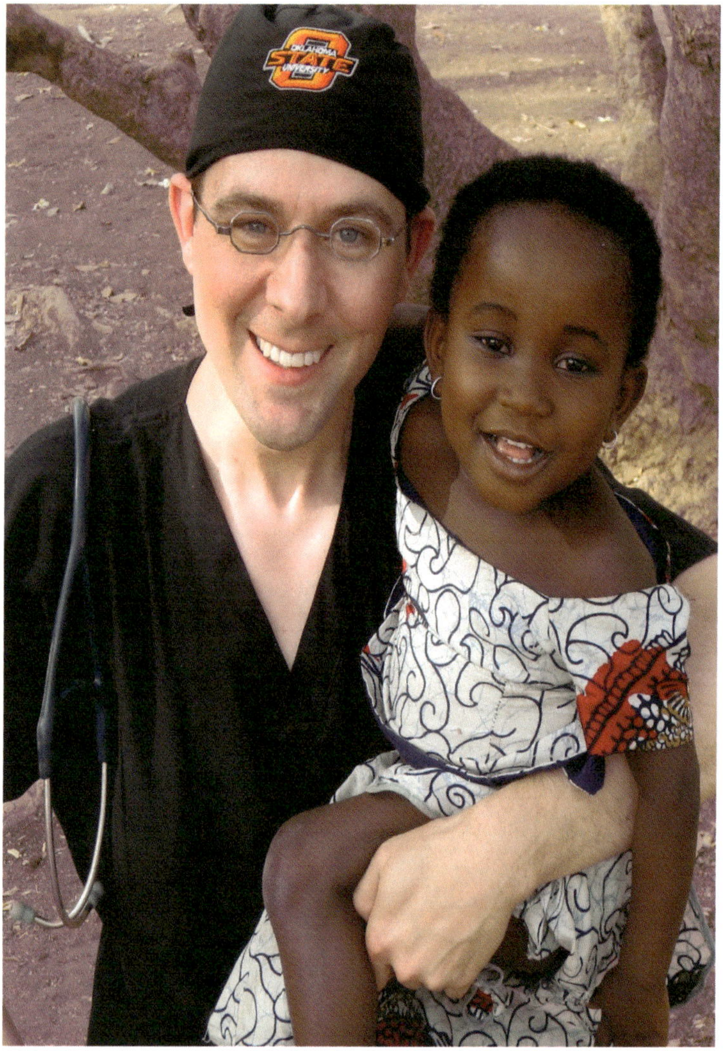

Love Is Also A Good Medicine.

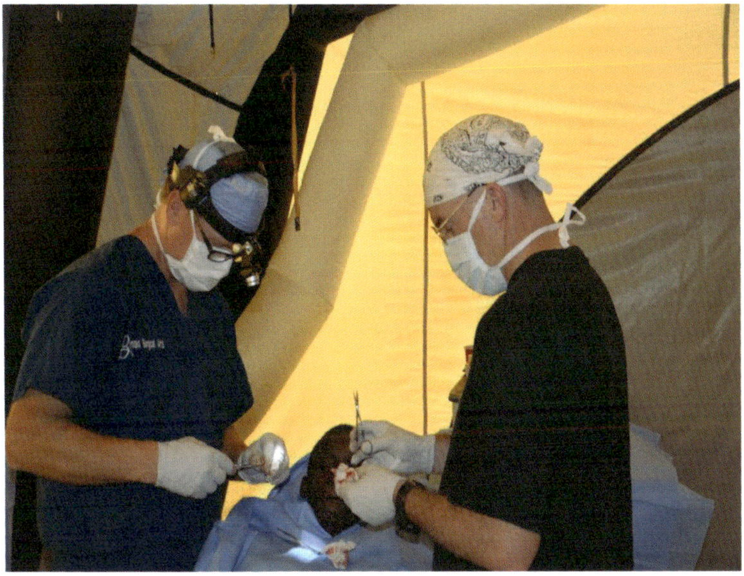

Medical Team Hard At Work

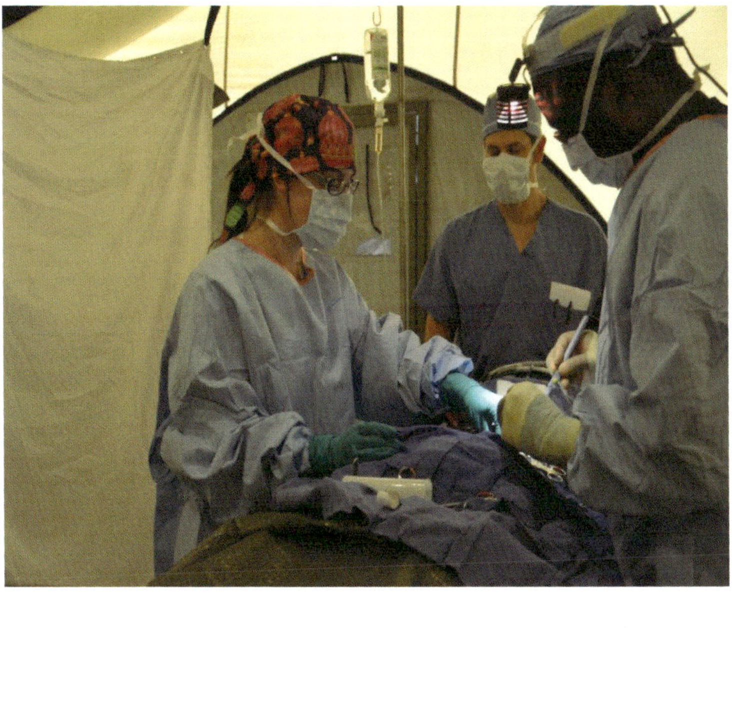

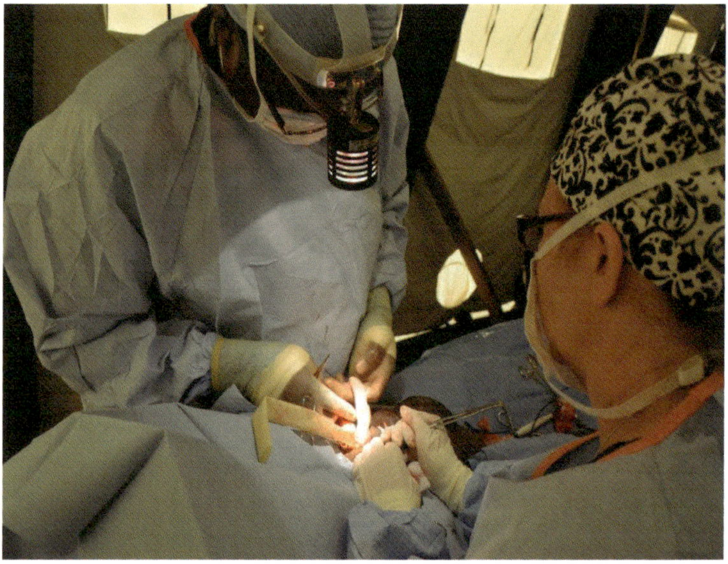

In The Field Or Hospital,
The Medical Team Was There To Help.

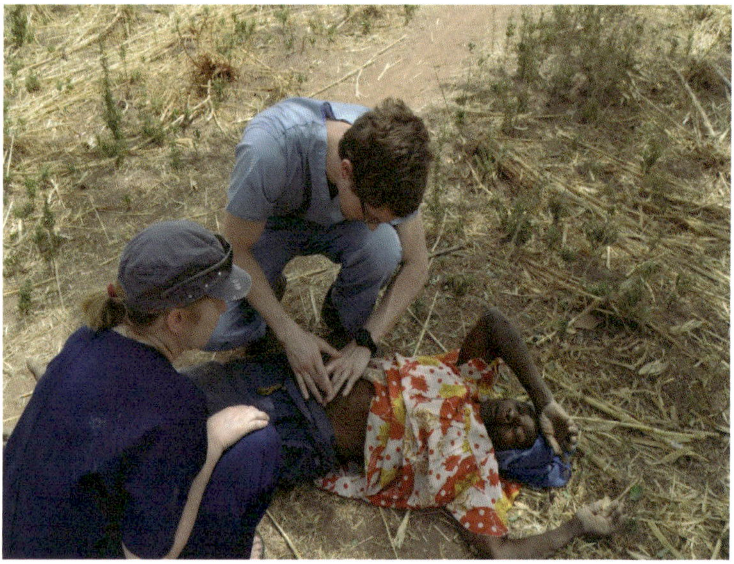

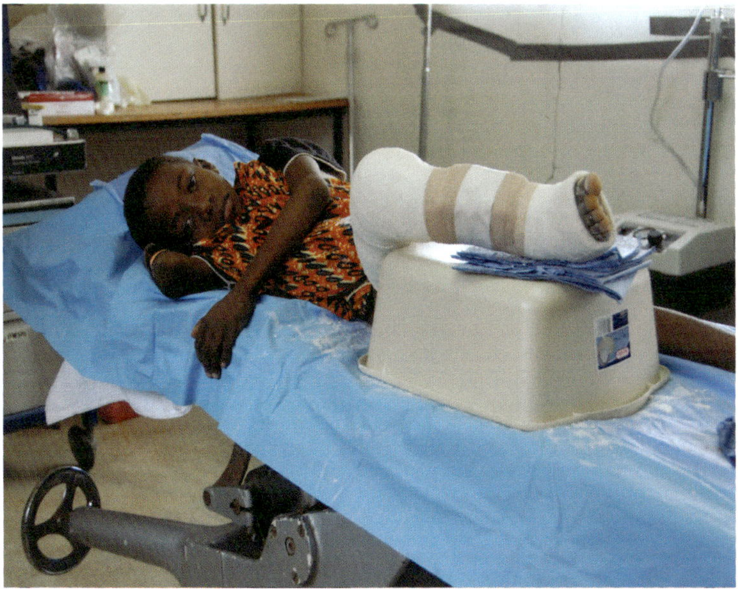

Repair Of A Fractured Leg.

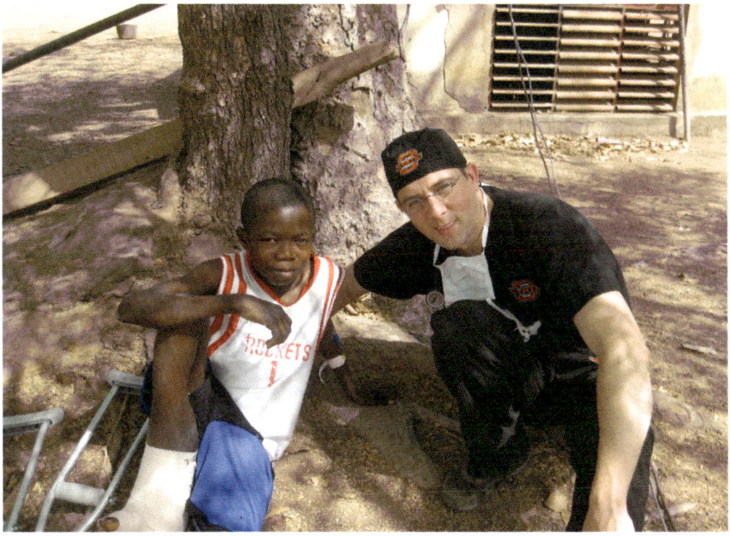

Simon, Who Had Extensive Foot Surgery, And Micah

If Feet Could Talk—

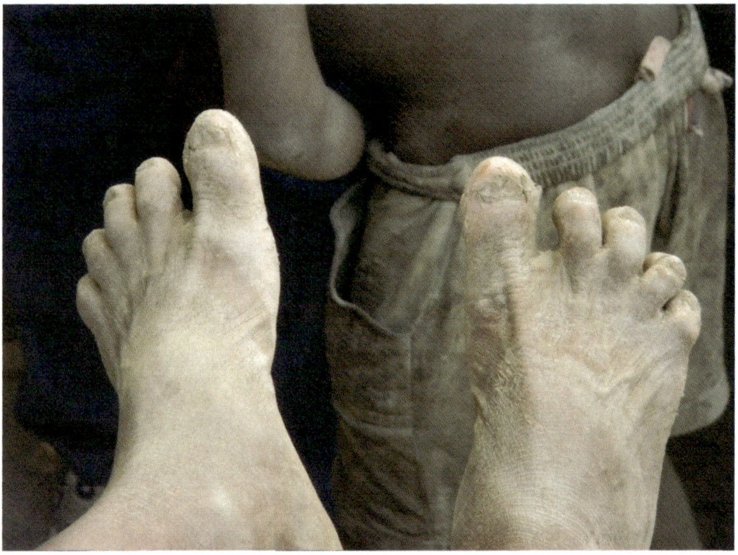

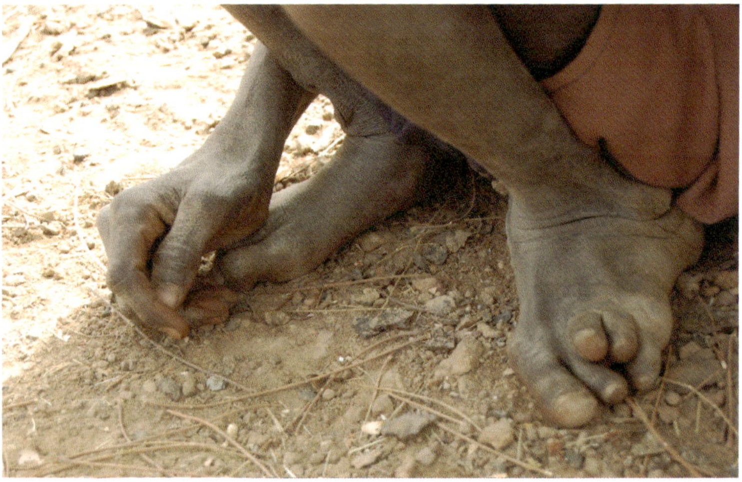

—What Would We Learn?

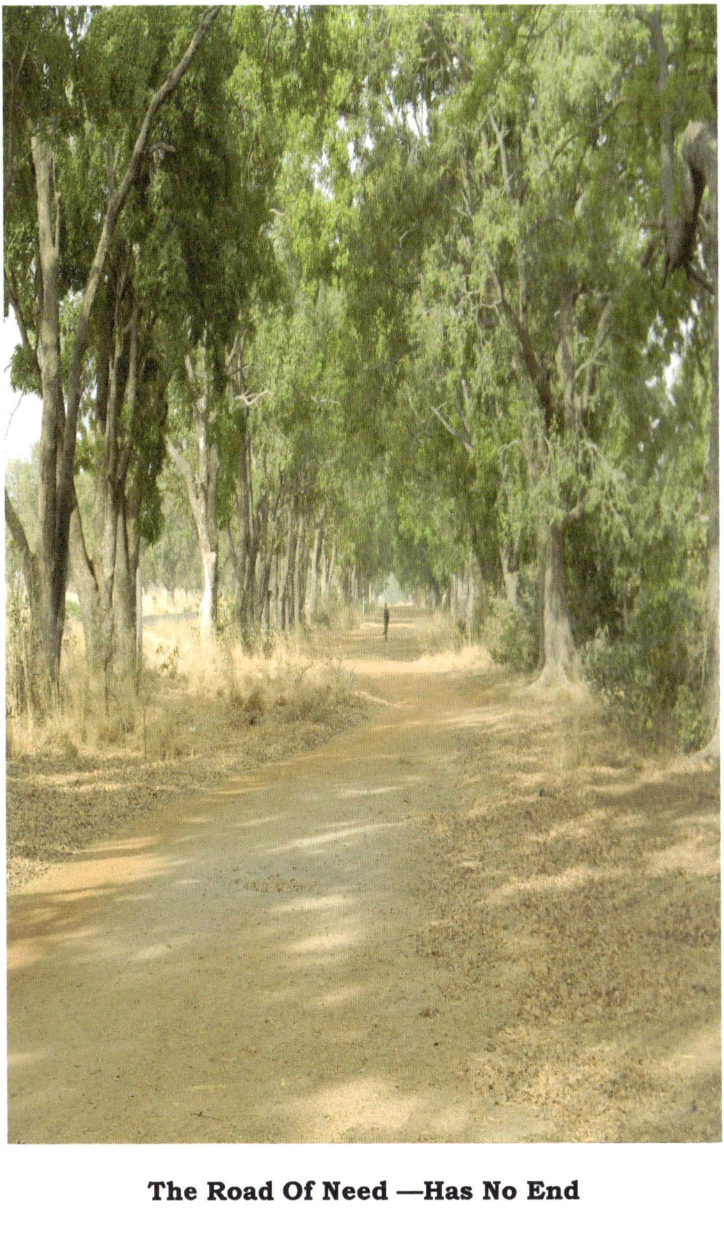

The Road Of Need —Has No End

GOD TRULY BLESSED AMERICA

As I reflected on the recent trip to "the uttermost parts," I asked myself what did I take away from the experience? What stood out more than anything else? Hopefully I was able to convey most of the highlights in my writings but there was one overwhelming truth I gleaned from the experience. It was the realization how blessed we are as a people and nation.

Throughout the 12 days spent in Africa, I heard many comments from the "campers" how unfair life seemed for the poor living in this part of the country. Their opinions came from personal awareness and hands on contact with the people. The environment truly is hostile to life in that it is easy to die from the most minor of things. Life threatening diseases, polio, tuberculosis, meningitis, cancer, HIV, and malaria are basically left untreated. Medical treatment is hard to come by and the quality of care certainly would not meet American standards. Education is scarce and any chance for self-improvement is limited. There are no sidewalks, paved streets, and modern day appliances or conveniences. Where would you put a washer and dryer in a mud hut without electricity or running water? There was nothing to help make life easy for man, woman, or child. Life was hard just to exist. Living required hard work.

I thought about this inequality often and concluded I am so happy to live in the United States of America but perhaps it is not for the reasons one might expect. The conveniences we enjoy make our lives easier and they are wonderful as are the freedoms to do whatever we want that is within the law. The one thing I am so grateful for is that our Founding Fathers had the foresight and sensibility to establish our country on the principles found in the Word of God. It is my opinion that our Founders' foresight and dependence on God prevented our country from being established as just another country—a country that might be socialist or communist; or one ruled by oppressive tyrants and dictators; or even an impoverished third world country.

George Washington felt that God ordained this country to be free and that God had called him to lead the fight for freedom. He even said that no human could create a free nation—only God could do that. Thomas Jefferson felt that without God, this nation would never have been formed. Although Abraham Lincoln was not a Founding Father, he said that we have been the recipients of the choicest bounties of Heaven. He knew that a Christian nation would receive only the best, the abundant blessings from God, and all knew the importance or significance God had played in establishing and maintaining a blessed, free nation.

We truly have enjoyed the blessings of God on this country. We are blessed because God's handprint was all over the Founding documents that govern our land—the Declaration of Independence and the Constitution. There has never been another country like the United States. We are who we are as a nation because of God. The Bible tells us that, "Blessed is the nation whose God is the Lord." (Ps 33:12) We have certainly been blessed.

As I continued to reflect on the blessings of God on our nation, I am saddened by the fact we have, as a nation, turned our back on God in many respects. This is just my opinion based upon the political climate that exists today and the laws that now govern our lives. Goodness is punished and evil is tolerated. Everything is all upside-down and our country is in serious trouble. We have forgotten what made it great. How much longer will God continue to bless our nation when we have tried to kick Him out of our homes, schools, and government? If this trend continues, will we forfeit our Christian heritage and crumble into an oppressive nation where freedoms are controlled by murderous regimes? Could it even be possible we could become a third world country that knows nothing but abject poverty and limited freedoms? Will people then come to help us construct buildings, dig wells, and offer medical care to our people? Will our children be allowed to live free or will they suffer by the stifling control of corrupted power?

There is a remedy to the infractions of our nation and its people that can be found in II Chronicles 7:14: “If my people who are called by My name will humble themselves, and pray and seek My face, and turn from their wicked ways, then I will hear from heaven, and will forgive their sin and heal their land.”

As my mind leaves the African continent and returns to America, I am made acutely aware of how fortunate we are to live in this wonderful country and how desperately I want God to heal our land. I want to continue to be a people living in a country blessed by God so that we can give abundantly to those who have not. I want to continue to have the freedom to take the Good News into villages darkened by centuries of idolatry. I want to remain free and live my freedom and faith by helping others and fulfilling God’s Great Commission. But how much longer will I be allowed to fulfill my heart’s desire? Liberty must be protected and preserved. It begins by returning to God and asking Him to heal—restore our country back to the country He intended for us to enjoy so that we may continue to impact a lost and dying world.

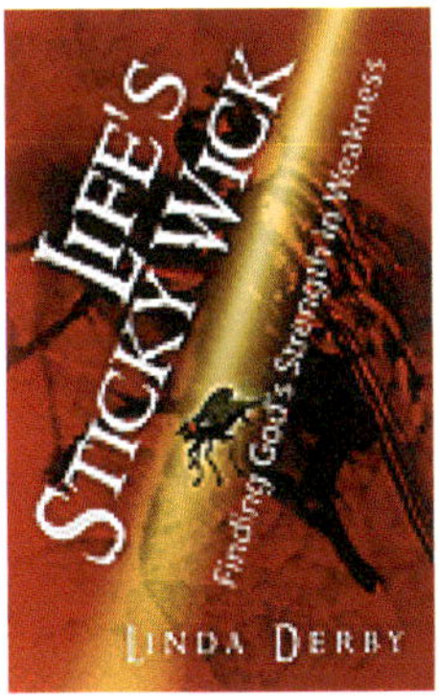

Linda Derby is an author, R. N., married, mother of three, and grandmother to seven. She has served in outreach ministries in her denomination for over 30 years and as a Christian educator for women of diverse cultures. Her articles have appeared in such publications as the denominational magazine, GEM, and the Rejoice Magazine.

She is the author of *His Story*, a biography of a World War II Prisoner of War hero, and is the co-author of *Bismarck: Hometown U.S.A.*, a history book about her hometown. Linda lives with her family in Owasso, Oklahoma.

About the Author When life becomes difficult, painful, or uncertain, action must be taken to avoid complete disaster or breakdown. *Life's Sticky Wick* chronicles the journey through the emotional and spiritual trials of a Christian mother when her young daughter-in-law is diagnosed with cancer. Experience the spiritual action required by the author to successfully conquer the impact of a devastating disease on a family member and enjoy the teachings from God acquired along the way.

Testimonials:

"Here is a story worth sharing about a life worth living and a God worth serving."

Rob Morgan, Author, writer,
Senior Pastor of The Donelson Fellowship, Nashville, TN.

"I like good writers and Linda Derby is a very good one. I also like missionary stories and this story was a touching story about her son and his wife who on their first furlough discovered the missionary wife had serious cancer. This story will make you rejoice as you find God's strength and blessing.

Dr. Alton Loveless, Retired Publisher

Available in Swahili and in Kindle editions
www.amazon.com ISBN 1450020615

CPSIA information can be obtained
at www.ICGtesting.com
Printed in the USA
LVIW020459100712
289451LV00003B

* 9 7 8 0 9 8 4 7 9 7 4 5 5 *